# Reactions to Aspirin and Other Non-steroidal Anti-inflammatory Drugs

*Editors*

DONALD D. STEVENSON
MAREK L. KOWALSKI

## IMMUNOLOGY AND ALLERGY CLINICS OF NORTH AMERICA

www.immunology.theclinics.com

*Consulting Editor*
RAFEUL ALAM

May 2013 • Volume 33 • Number 2

**ELSEVIER**

1600 John F. Kennedy Boulevard • Suite 1800 • Philadelphia, Pennsylvania, 19103-2899.
http://www.theclinics.com

IMMUNOLOGY AND ALLERGY CLINICS OF NORTH AMERICA Volume 33, Number 2
May 2013 ISSN 0889–8561, ISBN-13: 978-1-4557-4848-8

Editor: Pamela Hetherington

*Immunology and Allergy Clinics of North America* (ISSN 0889–8561) is published quarterly by Elsevier Inc., 360 Park Avenue South, New York, NY 10010-1710. Months of issue are February, May, August, and November. Periodicals postage paid at New York, NY and additional mailing offices. Subscription prices are $306.00 per year for US individuals, $442.00 per year for US institutions, $144.00 per year for US students and residents, $375.00 per year for Canadian individuals, $209.00 per year for Canadian students, $547.00 per year for Canadian institutions, $425.00 per year for international individuals, $547.00 per year for international institutions, $209.00 per year for international students. To receive student/resident rate, orders must be accompanied by name of affiliated institution, date of term, and the *signature* of program/residency coordinator on institution letterhead. Orders will be billed at individual rate until proof of status is received. Foreign air speed delivery is included in all *Clinics* subscription prices. All prices are subject to change without notice. **POSTMASTER**: Send address changes to *Immunology and Allergy Clinics of North America,* Elsevier Health Sciences Division, Subscription Customer Service, 3251 Riverport Lane, Maryland Heights, MO 63043. **Customer Service: 1-800-654-2452 (U.S. and Canada); 314-447-8871 (outside U.S. and Canada). Fax: 314-447-8029. E-mail: journalscustomerservice-usa@elsevier.com (for print support); journalsonlinesupport-usa@elsevier.com (for online support).**

*Reprints.* For copies of 100 or more, of articles in this publication, please contact the Commercial Reprints Department, Elsevier Inc., 360 Park Avenue South, New York, New York 10010-1710. Tel. (212) 633-3812, Fax: (212) 462-1935, E-mail: reprints@elsevier.com.

*Immunology and Allergy Clinics of North America is covered in MEDLINE/PubMed (Index Medicus), Current Contents/Life Sciences, Science Citation Index, ISI/BIOMED, Chemical Abstracts, and EMBASE/Excerpta Medica.*

Printed and bound by CPI Group (UK) Ltd, Croydon, CR0 4YY
Transferred to digital print 2013

# Contributors

## CONSULTING EDITOR

**RAFEUL ALAM, MD, PhD**
Professor and Chief, Division of Allergy and Immunology, National Jewish Health, University of Colorado Denver School of Medicine, Denver, Colorado

## EDITORS

**DONALD D. STEVENSON, MD**
Senior Consultant, Division of Allergy and Immunology, Scripps Clinic and the Scripps Research Institute, San Diego, California

**MAREK L. KOWALSKI, MD, PhD**
Professor and Chairman, Department of Immunology, Rheumatology and Allergy, Chair of Clinical Immunology and Microbiology, Medical University of Lodz, Łódź, Poland

## AUTHORS

**RAFEUL ALAM, MD, PhD**
Professor of Medicine, Director, Division of Allergy and Immunology, Veda and Chauncey Ritter Chair in Immunology, National Jewish Medical and Research Center, University of Colorado, Denver, Colorado

**GRAŻYNA BOCHENEK, MD, PhD**
Associate Professor, Department of Pulmonology, Jagiellonian University School of Medicine, Jagiellonian University Medical College, Krakow, Poland

**JOSHUA A. BOYCE, MD**
Brigham and Women's Hospital, Professor of Medicine, Harvard Medical School, Boston, Massachusetts

**TREVER BURNETT, MD**
Fellow, Adult Program, Department of Allergy and Immunology, National Jewish Medical and Research Center, University of Colorado, Denver, Colorado

**FERNAN CABALLERO-FONSECA, MD**
Department of Allergy and Clinical Immunology, Centro Médico-Docente La Trinidad, Caracas, Venezuela

**ARNALDO CAPRILES-HULETT, MD**
Department of Allergy and Clinical Immunology, Centro Médico-Docente La Trinidad, Caracas, Venezuela

**MARIANA CASTELLS, MD**
Director, Allergy and Clinical Immunology Training Program, Brigham and Women's Hospital; Professor of Medicine, Harvard Medical School, Boston, Massachusetts

**ROHIT KATIAL, MD, FAAAAI, FACP**
Professor of Medicine, Program Director, Weinberg Clinical Research Unit, Adult
Fellowship Program, Department of Allergy and Immunology, Director, National Jewish
Medical and Research Center, University of Colorado, Denver, Colorado

**SEUNG-HYUN KIM, PhD**
Associate Professor, Department of Allergy and Clinical Immunology, Ajou University
School of Medicine, Woncheondong, Youngtonggu, Suwon, Republic of Korea

**MAREK L. KOWALSKI, MD, PhD**
Professor and Chairman, Department of Immunology, Rheumatology and Allergy, Chair of
Clinical Immunology and Microbiology, Medical University of Lodz, Łodź, Poland

**TANYA M. LAIDLAW, MD**
Brigham and Women's Hospital, Instructor of Medicine, Harvard Medical School, Boston,
Massachusetts

**JOAQUIM MULLOL, MD, PhD**
Head, Rhinology Unit and Smell Clinic, Department of Otorhinolaryngology, Hospital
Clínic i Universitari, University of Barcelona, Catalonia, Spain; Clinical and Experimental
Respiratory Immunoallergy, Institut d'Investigacions Biomèdiques August Pi i Sunyer
(IDIBAPS); Centro de Investigación Biomédica en Red de Enfermedades Respiratorias
(CIBERES); Global Allergy and Asthma European Network (GA2LEN), Barcelona,
Catalonia, Spain

**EWA NIŻANKOWSKA-MOGILNICKA, MD, PhD, FCCP**
Professor, Head, Department of Pulmonology, Jagiellonian University School of
Medicine, Jagiellonian University Medical College, Skawińska, Krakow, Poland

**HAE-SIM PARK, MD, PhD**
Chairman, Professor, Department of Allergy and Clinical Immunology, Ajou University
School of Medicine, Woncheondong, Youngtonggu, Suwon, Republic of Korea

**CÉSAR PICADO, MD, PhD**
Clinical and Experimental Respiratory Immunoallergy, Institut d'Investigacions
Biomèdiques August Pi i Sunyer (IDIBAPS), Barcelona, Catalonia, Spain; Centro de
Investigación Biomédica en Red de Enfermedades Respiratorias (CIBERES); Global
Allergy and Asthma European Network (GA2LEN); Head, Allergy Unit, Department of
Pneumology and Respiratory Allergy, Hospital Clínic i Universitari, University of
Barcelona, Barcelona, Catalonia, Spain

**MARIO SÁNCHEZ-BORGES, MD**
Department of Allergy and Clinical Immunology, Centro Médico-Docente La Trinidad,
Caracas, Venezuela

**MAREK SANAK, MD, PhD**
Professor, Division of Molecular Biology and Clinical Genetics, Department of Medicine,
Jagiellonian University Medical College, Krakow, Poland

**RONALD A. SIMON, MD, FAAAAI**
Head, Division of Allergy, Asthma Immunology, Scripps Clinic, San Diego, California

**DONALD D. STEVENSON, MD**
Senior Consultant, Division of Allergy and Immunology, Scripps Clinic and the Scripps
Research Institute, San Diego, California

**ANDREW A. WHITE, MD**
Director of the Aspirin Desensitization Program, Member, Division of Allergy and Immunology, The Scripps Research Institute, Scripps Clinic, San Diego, California

**KATHARINE M. WOESSNER, MD, FAAAAI**
Program Director, Scripps Allergy and Immunology Fellowship Program, Division of Allergy and Immunology, Scripps Clinic, San Diego, California

# Contents

**Preface: A Dedication to Andrew Szczeklik, MD**                                        xi

Donald D. Stevenson and Marek L. Kowalski

**Introduction: Szczeklik's Contributions to Our Understanding of Aspirin, NSAIDs,
Asthma, and Allergy**                                                                   125

Donald D. Stevenson and Marek L. Kowalski

Andrew Szczeklik was born in 1938 and died on Feb 3rd, 2012. He was the most influential expert in the field of aspirin and NSAID sensitivity reactions and associated diseases in the world. This edition of NACAI is dedicated to Andrew. In the introductory chapter, we elected to highlight his accomplishments as reflected in his publications. Andrew published at least 503 articles including many invited review articles. We present 20 of his most important publications all of which contributed significantly to our understanding of these diseases.

**Classification of Reactions to Nonsteroidal Antiinflammatory Drugs**                   135

Marek L. Kowalski and Donald D. Stevenson

Hypersensitivity reactions to NSAIDs may occur in susceptible individuals and vary in symptom (skin, respiratory tract, and solid organs), severity (from mild skin or respiratory reactions to severe generalized) and timing (from acute to delayed). The current classification of NSAID-induced reactions emerged with the understanding of the pathologic mechanism of reactions to NSAIDs which may be either non-allergic (related to cyclo-oxygenase inhibition) or immunologically mediated. In this chapter we discuss the implications of accurate NSAIDs hypersensitivity classification for proper diagnosis and patient management.

**Aspirin-Exacerbated Respiratory Disease: Clinical Disease and Diagnosis**              147

Grażyna Bochenek and Ewa Niżankowska-Mogilnicka

This article summarizes the current knowledge in the field of clinical presentation and diagnosis of aspirin-exacerbated respiratory disease (AERD). The definition, prevalence, natural history, and clinical presentation of this distinct clinical syndrome are described. The classification and tolerance of particular groups of cyclooxygenase inhibitors by patients with AERD are presented. The authors comprehensively discuss provocation tests with aspirin as the most reliable method to confirm the diagnosis of AERD.

**Rhinosinusitis and Nasal Polyps in Aspirin-Exacerbated Respiratory Disease**           163

Joaquim Mullol and César Picado

The presence of aspirin-exacerbated respiratory disease (AERD) in a patient with chronic rhinosinusitis with nasal polyps and asthma is associated with severe eosinophilic upper and lower airway disease. This article deals with the inflammatory disease of the respiratory tract as it relates to the sinuses. Involvement of the sinuses in AERD is almost universal, depending on the stage of onset of the disease and evaluation by computed tomography. This article explores the clinical aspects, physiopathology, and treatment of rhinosinusitis as it relates to AERD.

## Genetics of Hypersensitivity to Aspirin and Nonsteroidal Anti-inflammatory Drugs    177

Seung-Hyun Kim, Marek Sanak, and Hae-Sim Park

Various hypersensitivity reactions have been reported with aspirin and nonsteroidal anti-inflammatory drugs. Hypersensitivity can occur regardless of a chemical drug structure or its therapeutic potency. Allergic conditions include aspirin-exacerbated respiratory disease (AERD or aspirin-induced asthma), aspirin-induced urticaria/angioedema (AIU), and anaphylaxis. Several genetic studies on aspirin hypersensitivity have been performed to discover the genetic predisposition to aspirin hypersensitivity and to gain insight into the phenotypic diversity. This article updates data on the genetic mechanisms that govern AERD and AIU and summarizes recent findings on the molecular genetic mechanism of aspirin hypersensitivity.

## Pathogenesis of Aspirin-Exacerbated Respiratory Disease and Reactions    195

Tanya M. Laidlaw and Joshua A. Boyce

Physiologic and pharmacologic studies support the hypothesis that aspirin-exacerbated respiratory disease (AERD) involves fundamental dysregulation in the production of and end-organ responsiveness to both antiinflammatory eicosanoids (prostaglandin $E_2$) and proinflammatory effectors (cysteinyl leukotrienes). The acquired nature of AERD implies a disturbance in a potential epigenetic control mechanism of the relevant mediator systems, which may be a result of incompletely clarified environmental factors (eg, viral or bacterial infections, inhaled pollutants).

## Aspirin Desensitization in Aspirin-Exacerbated Respiratory Disease    211

Andrew A. White and Donald D. Stevenson

Although aspirin desensitization was discovered in 1922, it was not until 1979 that a therapeutic use for aspirin treatment, under the protection of desensitization, was discovered. In the last 33 years, details of aspirin treatment have been refined to the point where it is now recognized and accepted as a major therapeutic intervention in the treatment of aspirin-exacerbated respiratory disease, with therapeutic efficacy in approximately two-thirds of patients. It is only effective in patients who have aspirin-exacerbated respiratory disease and none of the other nonsteroidal anti-inflammatory drugs, despite their cross-reactive inhibition of cyclooxygenase-1, can effectively take the place of aspirin.

## Mechanisms of Aspirin Desensitization    223

Trever Burnett, Rohit Katial, and Rafeul Alam

Aspirin-exacerbated respiratory disease is a clinical syndrome characterized by severe, persistent asthma, hyperplastic eosinophilic sinusitis with

nasal polyps, and reactions to aspirin and other nonsteroidal antiinflammatory drugs that preferentially inhibit cyclooxygenase 1. The mechanisms
behind the therapeutic effects of aspirin desensitization remain poorly
understood. Recent studies suggest that the clinical benefits may occur
through direct inhibition of tyrosine kinases and the signal transducer
and activator of transcription 6 signaling pathway, which results in inhibition of interleukin 4 production. In this article, the current understanding
of the mechanisms of aspirin desensitization is reviewed and future areas
of investigation are discussed.

## NSAID Single-Drug–Induced Reactions                        237

Katharine M. Woessner and Mariana Castells

Nonsteroidal anti-inflammatory drugs (NSAIDs) are cyclooxygenase inhibitors with analgesic, anti-inflammatory, antipyretic, and antithrombotic effects. NSAIDs have been implicated in a variety of drug-induced reactions
that are proved as or suspected of being mediated through a host immune
response. Single-drug–induced reactions are the hallmark of these types
of reactions. The types of single-drug–induced reactions are the confluence of 2 variables, the structure of the drug and the specific types of immune responses. This article identifies reactions patterns and the NSAIDs
most likely to elicit each immune response.

## Aspirin-Exacerbated Cutaneous Disease                      251

Mario Sánchez-Borges, Fernan Caballero-Fonseca, and Arnaldo Capriles-Hulett

It has been recognized that a high proportion of chronic urticaria patients
experience symptom aggravation when exposed to aspirin and NSAIDs.
This clinical picture is known as Aspirin-exacerbated cutaneous disease.
The pathogenesis of these exacerbations is related to the inhibition of
cyclooxygenase-1 leading to a decreased synthesis of PGE2 and an increased cysteinyl leukotriene production in the skin and subcutaneous
tissues. Patient management comprises the treatment of the underlying
cutaneous disease with nonsedating antihistamines and other medications, avoidance of COX-1 inhibitors, and the use of alternative NSAIDs
that do not inhibit COX-1 for the relief of pain, inflammation and fever.

## Cardiovascular Prophylaxis and Aspirin "Allergy"           263

Katharine M. Woessner and Ronald A. Simon

Aspirin is an important antiplatelet agent in the treatment of cardiovascular
disease. Aspirin "allergy" often directs the physician away from this
potentially life-saving modality. The majority of patients with a history of
"reactions to aspirin" have aspirin/nonsteroidal anti-inflammatory drug
(NSAID)-induced gastritis, easy bruisability, or other side effects. The minority of these patients has a "true allergy," referred to as a hypersensitivity
reaction. The former group can be started on aspirin without the need for
special challenge. Adding a proton-pump inhibitor can often mitigate the
gastrointestinal side effects. Patients with aspirin hypersensitivity can be
safely challenged with aspirin.

**Index**                                                     275

# IMMUNOLOGY AND ALLERGY
# CLINICS OF NORTH AMERICA

## FORTHCOMING ISSUES

**August 2013**
Exercise-Induced Bronchospasm
Sandra Anderson, *Editor*

**November 2013**
Angioedema
Bruce Zuraw, *Editor*

**February 2014**
Urticaria
Malcolm Greaves, *Editor*

### ISSUE OF RELATED INTEREST

*Clinics in Chest Medicine* June 2012 (Volume 33, Number 2)
**Bronchiectasis**
Mark L. Metersky, MD, and Anne E. O'Donnell, MD, *Editors*

# Preface

# A Dedication to Andrew Szczeklik, MD

This issue of *Allergy and Immunology Clinics of North America* is in memory of our friend and colleague, Andrew Szczeklik. Those of us who had the pleasure of knowing this wonderful physician and scientist will remember him for many things: friendships, combined projects, discoveries, discussions, and active collaborations with many scientists around the world. This issue focuses on Andrew's life passion, namely, the questions about why aspirin and other nonsteroidal anti-inflammatory drugs (NSAIDs) behave in such peculiar ways when compared to other drug molecules. The mixture of pharmacologic pseudo-allergic effects and specific stimulation of key parts of the immune system that generate allergic reactions is truly unique among medications used by humans. Andrew was, from the beginning of this quest, a driving force in answering most of these basic and clinical questions. Indeed, the 2 guest editors cannot think of any investigator in the past 40 years that has contributed more to this field of science than Andrew Szczeklik.

Our goal, in putting together this issue, was to explore all aspects of aspirin and other NSAID-induced reactions. We are convinced that the articles in this issue and the list of outstanding contributors who produced these articles have provided the reader with everything that is currently known about this subject. Anyone who knew Andy or read his many contributions in this field can see Andrew's observations and discoveries sprinkled throughout all these articles. Indeed, we were so struck by this observation that we converted the introduction article into a celebration of Andrew's life and included within it 20 peer-reviewed articles by Andrew and coauthors. This is fascinating reading by itself but it also supports our thesis that Andrew Szczeklik was in the middle of this area of Allergy Discovery over the past 40 years. As you read our introductory article of this issue, such conclusions become obvious.

Our introduction also focuses on Andrew as the humanitarian. As scientists, we are focused on his products of scientific investigations and publications. But more than that, Andrew was a humanitarian of the very best type. He always praised others for their efforts. He did everything he could to bring scientists together with mutual investigations and transfer of information. He set up conferences on these subjects and had letter correspondence and then e-mail interactions with interested scientists throughout the world. He was generous with his ideas and encouraged everyone, but particularly younger colleagues, to step up to the next level of investigations. Even in the 1970s, he was very thoughtful about where this field was going and quite early concluded that aspirin-induced asthma was only partially genetic and that an environmental insult, which he very early on predicted was a viral respiratory infection, was needed to complete the dysfunction that leads to the inflammatory respiratory disease. He and his colleagues discovered similar mechanisms in the cutaneous variant, namely, chronic idiopathic urticaria.

Immunol Allergy Clin N Am 33 (2013) xi–xii
http://dx.doi.org/10.1016/j.iac.2012.12.004
0889-8561/13/$ – see front matter © 2013 Published by Elsevier Inc.

immunology.theclinics.com

For the 2 guest editors, this was a labor of love. We thank consulting editor Rafeul Alam for inviting us to be guest editors and most of all for the privilege of being able to share with the entire world what Andrew meant to us and to many of you. Aspirin is no longer a mystery drug. Thank you, Andy, for what you have done for mankind.

Donald D. Stevenson, MD
Scripps Clinic and the Scripps Research Institute
3811 Valley Center Drive
San Diego, CA 92037, USA

Marek L. Kowalski, MD, PhD
Department of Immunology, Rheumatology & Allergy, Medical University of Lodz
251 Pomorska Street, Blg 5
92-213 Łódź, Poland

E-mail addresses:
Stevenson.donald@scrippshealth.org (D.D. Stevenson)
Marek.Kowalski@csk.umed.lodz.pl (M.L. Kowalski)

# Introduction
## Szczeklik's Contributions to Our Understanding of Aspirin, NSAIDs, Asthma, and Allergy

Donald D. Stevenson, MD[a],*, Marek L. Kowalski, MD, PhD[b]

### KEYWORDS

- Szczeklik • Aspirin • NSAIDs • AERD • Urticaria

### KEY POINTS

- Andrew Szczeklik contributed 503 medical articles during his lifetime.
- We selected 20 articles that contributed to our growing fund of knowledge in the area of drug hypersensitivity, particularly NSAIDs.

Born in 1938, 1 year before the Nazi invasion of Poland and growing up in post–World War II communist Poland, Andy Szczeklik not only survived the considerable difficulties imposed on Poland and all its citizens by these repressive governments but also rose to the top of the international medical community in patient care, teaching, administrative excellence, and both basic and translational research. In addition to his productive research and extensive publications, he skillfully chaired the Department of Medicine, Jagiellonian University Medical School, Krakow, Poland, for more than 40 years.

The number of Andy's friends are so numerous that selecting authors for this edition of the *Immunology and Allergy Clinics of North America* became an impossible task. We simply did not have enough articles or space to invite all of his many collaborators to participate as authors. We hope that those not invited will understand and, with the same gentle spirit that Andy approached all of us, will read and treasure this issue as a remembrance of Andy. With these thoughts in mind, this issue of the *Immunology and Allergy Clinics of North America* is dedicated to Andrew Szczeklik, a remarkable physician scientist.

Andy was an author or coauthor of 499 peer-reviewed scientific journal articles as recorded in PubMed. Again, space does not allow honoring all of these contributions and the many coauthors who would enjoy reading and remembering their studies or

Disclosures: None.
[a] Division of Allergy and Immunology, Scripps Research Institute, Scripps Clinic, 3811 Valley Center Drive, San Diego, CA 92130, USA; [b] Department of Immunology, Rheumatology and Allergy, Medical University of Lodz, Lodz, Poland
* Corresponding author.
*E-mail addresses:* dstevensonmd@gmail.com; stevenson.donald@scrippshealth.org

Immunol Allergy Clin N Am 33 (2013) 125–133
http://dx.doi.org/10.1016/j.iac.2012.10.001
0889-8561/13/$ – see front matter © 2013 Elsevier Inc. All rights reserved.

immunology.theclinics.com

reviews that were conducted with Andy. Publications that were pivotal in moving knowledge forward, however, and were specifically directed at aspirin-exacerbated respiratory disease (AERD), urticaria, or nonsteroidal anti-inflammatory drug (NSAID) reactions were selected by the guest editors for remembrance of this great man. Highlighted publications and our comments about these 20 major contributions are as follows.

1. **Szczeklik A**, Gryglewski RJ, Czerniawska-Mysik G. Relationship of inhibition of prostaglandin biosynthesis by analgesics to asthma attacks in aspirin-sensitive patients. Br Med J 1975;1:67–9.

This classic study, published in January 1975, when Andrew was 37 years old, is a landmark investigation in the pathogenesis of reactions to aspirin and other NSAIDs in patients with AERD. It changed the entire direction of understanding of aspirin-induced respiratory reactions. For the first time, Andrew and his colleagues showed that drugs (NSAIDs) that inhibited microsomal prostaglandin synthetase in vitro (aspirin, indomethacin, mefenamic acid, flufenamic acid, and phenylbutazone) also induced asthma attacks during oral challenges in 11 sensitive asthmatics. By contrast, therapeutic doses of salicylamide, parcetamol, benzydamine, and chloroquine, which did not inhibit prostaglandin synthetase, did not induce asthma attacks in the same 11 patients. The previously unknown mechanism of cross-reactions between aspirin and other NSAIDs, originally demonstrated by Professor Fernand Widal in 1922 and then Professor Max Samter in 1967, was now shown to be a shared pharmacologic effect, namely inhibition of cyclooxygenase (COX) enzymes.

2. **Szczeklik A**, Gryglewski RJ, Czerniawska-Mysik G, Zmuda A. Aspirin-induced asthma. Hypersensitivity to fenoprofen and ibuprofen in relation to their inhibitory action on prostaglandin generation by different microsomal enzymic preparations. J Allergy Clin Immunol 1976;58:10–8.

Using 3 known NSAIDS, aspirin, fenoprofen, and ibuprofen, Andrew and colleagues were able to correlate provoking doses of these 3 NSAIDs, as shown during oral challenges in aspirin-sensitive asthmatics, with the degree of inhibition of prostaglandins in vitro, using bovine seminal vesicles, rabbit brain, and rabbit kidney medulla. As a control, dextropropxyphene did not inhibit prostaglandin synthesis nor did it induce asthmatic reactions in the study asthmatics. This was the first study to demonstrate that the dose response for each NSAID was different and could be predicted from the in vitro dose needed to inhibit prostaglandin synthesis in vitro. Furthermore, a certain challenge dose (threshold dose) had to be reached before an asthmatic reaction was induced.

3. **Szczeklik A**, Gryglewski RJ, Olszewski E, Dembińska-Kiec A, Czerniawska-Mysik G. Aspirin-sensitive asthma: the effect of aspirin on the release of prostaglandins from nasal polyps. Pharmacol Res Commun 1977;9:415–25.

Using bioassay to detect prostaglandin-like material (prostaglandin E2 [$PGE_2$]) in nasal polyp pieces and homogenates, Andy and his coauthors demonstrated that aspirin more effectively inhibited prostaglandin biosynthesis in tissues derived from aspirin-sensitive patients than in nonsensitive control asthmatics. This early study discovered that the cellular enzyme system generating PGE in aspirin-sensitive patients had an increased susceptibility to the inhibitory action of aspirin. They provided this early experimental evidence that the prostaglandin (arachidonic acid metabolism) systems itself was implicated in the pathologic susceptibility to NSAIDs hypersensitivity in patients with AERD.

4. **Szczeklik A**, Gryglewski RJ, Czerniawska-Mysik G. Participation of prostaglandins in pathogenesis of aspirin-sensitive asthma. Naunyn Schmiedebergs Arch Pharmacol 1977;297(Suppl 1):S99–110.

"Recent evidence suggests that the induction of bronchoconstriction in aspirin-sensitive patients by analgesics is due to the inhibition of PG biosynthesis in their respiratory tract. PGEs might play the main defensive role in the bronchi of aspirin-sensitive asthmatics. Removal of this potent bronchodilator by PG synthetase inhibitors leaves the effects of spasmogens unopposed, and possibly promotes the release of histamine from its stores." This was the first published theory that described the mechanism by which inhibition of COX could block PGE synthesis, reduce its preventive effects on inflammation, and thus release the pent up inflammatory cascade, which occurs during NSAID reactions in patients with AERD. The authors also predicted that another "spasmogen" (ie, soon to be discovered in 1979 as cysteinyl-leukotriene [cys-LTs]) were also prevented from activation by PGE.

5. **Szczeklik A**, Serwonska M. Inhibition of idiosyncratic reactions to aspirin in asthmatic patients by clemastine. Thorax 1979;34:654–7.

Clemastine, an $H_1$ receptor blocking antihistamine, when taken before oral aspirin challenges, prevented flushing, rhinorrhea, cough, and headache in 10 aspirin-sensitive asthmatics who underwent standard oral aspirin challenges. Although effective in blocking some of the upper airway responses and extrapulmonary reactions during oral aspirin challenges, this antihistamine had only partial modifying effects on asthmatic responses to aspirin. This suggested that "other spasmogens" were also inducing bronchoconstriction in aspirin-sensitive asthmatics. A role for histamine release as a part of the aspirin-induced respiratory reactions was clearly implied in this early study.

6. Czerniawska-Mysik G, **Szczeklik A**. Idiosyncrasy to pyrazolone drugs. Allergy 1981;36:381–4.

In 68 patients, all NSAIDs induced hives or asthma. The weak pyrazolones, oramidopyrine and aminophenazone, however, did not induce any reactions in this selected group of 68 patients. But the same drugs induced anaphylactic shock and/or urticaria in a second group of historically sensitive patients. Skin tests with these drugs induced positive wheal and flare reactions in this second group of sensitive patients. Phenylbutazone, sulfinpyrazone, and aspirin could be taken without inducing any reactions in this second group of patients. Andrew and colleagues suggested that the pathogenic mechanisms responsible for the idiosyncratic reactions involve either inhibition of COX, which was the mechanism in the first group, and true IgE-mediated allergic reactions in the second group. Thus, pyrazolones participated in IgE-mediated reactions, which are drug specific and not subject to cross-reactivity.

7. **Szczeklik A**. Analgesics, allergy and asthma. Drugs 1986;32(Suppl 4):148–63.

This classic early review article highlighted the different mechanisms by which the same NSAIDs could participate in reactions. The underlying clinical disease of a patient largely determined the type of adverse response to an analgesic. Up to 40% of patients with chronic urticaria develop an obvious increase in urticaria and angioedema after taking aspirin. In certain normal-appearing individuals, analgesics can produce anaphylactic reactions and/or urticaria to single NSAIDs, whereas in some asthmatics, NSAIDs precipitate bronchoconstriction. Mechanisms seem to be either IgE mediated and COX blockade for anaphylaxis and urticarial reactions and only

COX blockade for asthmatic reactions. Thus, the same analgesics can participate in at least 2 different types of reaction mechanisms that induce urticarial reactions but bronchospastic reactions are only mediated by COX blockade and depletion of $PGE_2$.

8. **Szczeklik A**. Aspirin-induced asthma as a viral disease. Clin Allergy 1988;18:15–20.

Andrew was the first investigator to make the observation that aspirin-induced asthma (AIA) frequently started shortly after a viral respiratory infection. The concept that otherwise healthy patients, or those with mild allergic rhinitis, developed a cold and never recover, was Andrew's theory that AERD was a combination of a genetic predisposition whose phenotype required an external assault, such as a viral respiratory infection, before the disease could begin. Once started, AERD could then self-perpetuate.

9. Sladek K, **Szczeklik A**. Cysteinyl leukotrienes overproduction and mast cell activation in aspirin-provoked bronchospasm in asthma. Eur Respir J 1993;6:391–9.

In 10 AIA patients, urinary leukotriene $E_4$ ($uLTE_4$) excretion was increased 7-fold 4 to 6 hours after aspirin challenge, whereas 11-dehydrothromboxane $B_2$ ($11\text{-}dTXB_2$), a downstream prostanoid of COX-1 synthesis, decreased gradually, reaching 50% baseline levels 24 hours after challenge ($P<.05$). The levels of both increasing $LTE_4$ and decreasing $11\text{-}dTXB_2$ responses depended on the dose of aspirin used in the challenges ($P<.001$, analysis of variance). They also measured serum tryptase and eosinophil cationic protein (ECP) levels as evidence of activation of mast cells and eosinophils. Thus, the correlation with a documented bronchospastic response to aspirin with a decline in a COX-1 products and a surge in leukotrienes was established. Mast cells and eosinophils had to be participating cells in the bronchospastic reactions.

10. **Szczeklik A**, Sladek K, Dworski R, Nizankowska E, Soja J, Sheller J, Oates J. Bronchial aspirin challenge causes specific eicosanoid response in aspirin-sensitive asthmatics. Am J Respir Crit Care Med 1996;154:1608–14.

Eleven asthmatics with AIA and 14 asthmatics, tolerant to aspirin (aspirin-tolerant asthma [ATA]), underwent bronchoalveolar lavage (BAL) after instillation of saline followed immediately by instillation of 10 mg of lysine aspirin, into a right middle lobe segmental bronchus. At baseline, the 2 groups did not differ with respect to BAL fluid concentrations of COX products, peptido-leukotrienes, histamine, tryptase, interleukin-5 (IL-5), eosinophil cationic protein (ECP), or numbers of eosinophils. Fifteen minutes after aspirin instillation, BAL fluid contained a significant rise in peptido-leukotrienes, IL-5, and numbers of eosinophils in AIA patients but not in ATA patients. Mean histamine concentrations rose in 7 of 11 AIA patients after acetylsalicylate (ASA) lysine, approaching statistical significance. Tryptase and ECP levels showed no significant changes in this early sample. This complicated study only use 1 provoking dose of ASA lysine, thus dose-dependent stimulation of histamine could not occur, and only 1 BAL sample at 15 minutes, eliminating late measurement of tryptase and ECP. Aspirin significantly depressed $PGE_2$ and $TXB_2$ in both groups. This was the first study to demonstrate disappearance of $PGE_2$ in the bronchi during topical bronchial challenge with aspirin lysine, occurring precisely at the time that inflammatory mediators were released or generated.

11. Cowburn AS, Sladek K, Soja J, Adamek L, Nizankowska E, **Szczeklik A**, Lam BK, Penrose JF, Austen FK, Holgate ST, Sampson AP. Over expression of leukotriene

C4 synthase in bronchial biopsies from patients with aspirin-intolerant asthma. J Clin Invest 1998;101:834–46.

To investigate why aspirin does not cause bronchoconstriction in all individuals, immunostained enzymes of the leukotriene and prostanoid pathway enzymes in bronchial biopsies from AIA patients, ATA patients, and normal (N) subjects were identified. Counts of cells expressing the terminal enzyme for cys-LT synthesis, leukotriene C4 synthase (LTC$_4$S), were 5-fold higher in AIA biopsies (11.5 ± 2.2 cells/mm$^2$, n = 10) than in ATA biopsies (2.2 ± 0.7, n = 10; $P$ = .0006) and 18-fold higher than in N biopsies (0.6 ± 0.4, n = 9; $P$ = .0002). Immunostaining for 5-lipoxygenase, its activating protein (FLAP), LTA$_4$ hydrolase, COX-1, and COX-2 did not differ. Enhanced baseline cys-LT levels in BAL fluid of AIA patients correlated uniquely with bronchial counts of LTC$_4$S positive cells (rho = 0.83, $P$ = .01). Lysine-aspirin challenges released additional cys-LTs into BAL fluid in AIA patients (200 ± 120 pg/mL, n = 8) but not in ATA patients (0. 7 ± 5.1, n = 5; $P$ = .007). Bronchial responsiveness to lysine-aspirin correlated exclusively with LTC$_4$S-positive cell counts (rho = −0.63, $P$ = .049, n = 10). Aspirin may remove PGE$_2$-dependent inflammatory suppression in all subjects, but only in AIA patients did increased bronchial expression of LTC$_4$S encourage marked overproduction of cys-LTs and bronchoconstriction.

12. Milewski M, Mastalerz L, Nizankowska E, **Szczeklik A**. Nasal provocation test with lysine-aspirin for diagnosis of aspirin-sensitive asthma. J Allergy Clin Immunol 1998;101:581–6.

Fifty-one patients with AIA, confirmed by oral aspirin challenge tests, were recruited to undergo diagnostic nasal inhalation challenge tests with lysine-aspirin. In 10 of these patients (19.6%), nasal provocation test could not be performed because of total obstruction of at least one nostril or marked fluctuations in nasal flow rates, leaving 41 patients with AIA for the study. The control groups consisted of 13 ATA patients and 10 healthy subjects. Polylysine-acetyl salicylic acid (L-ASA) at a total dose of 16 mg of acetylsalicylic acid was applied bilaterally into the inferior nasal turbinates. This caused a significant fall in inspiratory nasal flow in at least one nostril (>40%), measured by anterior rhinomanometry and clinical symptoms of watery discharge and nasal blockage in 35 of 41 patients with AIA, 1 of 10 healthy subjects, and none of 13 ATA patients. No systemic reactions or bronchospasm were noticed. This test was highly specific (95.7%) and sensitive (86.7%), but negative results did not exclude intolerance to aspirin (predictive value of a negative result 78.6%). Patients suspected of aspirin intolerance, who have a negative L-ASA test, should then undergo bronchial or oral challenge tests with aspirin.

13. **Szczeklik A**, NNizankowska E, Duplaga M. Natural history of aspirin-induced asthma: AIANE Investigators. European Network on Aspirin-Induced Asthma. Eur Respir J 2000;16:432–6.

This was a major collaborative study of European centers that were studying AIA. It illustrates Andy's leadership in bringing together researchers and their patient populations from 16 European centers in 10 countries, all of whom were tracking AIA. Because of the size of the study group, 500 patients, the investigators were able to make several important observations and characteristics of AIA, such as onset of aspirin disease at age 29, female preponderance 2.3 to 1, and a 15% incidence of patients who were unaware of having the disease until undergoing diagnostic oral aspirin challenges. In addition, the severity of AIA was established, in that 51% of the patients were taking continuous systemic corticosteroids, at a mean dose of 8 mg of prednisone per day, to control their disease.

14. Nizankowska E, Bestyńska-Krypel A, Cmiel A, **Szczeklik A**. Oral and bronchial provocation tests with aspirin for diagnosis of aspirin-induced asthma. Eur Respir J 2000;15:863–9.

In 35 asthmatic patients with suspected, by historical description and some with prior positive oral aspirin challenges, of having AIA and 15 asthmatics tolerating ASA, based on histories, the investigators compared the diagnostic value of placebo-controlled oral ASA challenge versus inhaled L-lysine–ASA challenges. Doses of ASA, increasing in geometric progression, were used in oral tests 10 mg to 312 mg (cumulative dose 500 mg), in bronchial tests 0.18 mg to 115 mg (cumulative dose 182 mg). A challenge was considered positive (ie, diagnostic of AERD) if the forced expiratory volume in the first second of expiration ($FEV_1$) dropped at least 20% from the baseline value and/or strong extrabronchial symptoms occurred (ie, nasal ocular reactions). $uLTE_4$ excretion was measured at baseline and after the challenges. In 24 of 35 patients, the oral ASA challenge test was positive, based on a 20% decrease in FEV1. When including extrabronchial symptoms, this was positive in 31 of 35 patients. Bronchial L-ASA challenges led to greater than or equal to or 20% fall FEV1 in 21 out of 35 cases and in 27 of 35 cases when including extrabronchial symptoms. In other words, 4 patients with nasal ocular reactions during oral aspirin challenge would have been misdiagnosed as negative, if only bronchial inhalation challenge was used. Stimulation of only the bronchial tissues with L-ASA, however, nevertheless generated nasal, ocular, and systemic reactions in some patients No correlation was observed between ASA provocative dose causing a 20% fall in $FEV_1$, determined by the oral route compared with the inhalation route. $uLTE_4$ increased after both challenges, the rise being higher after oral compared with inhalation L-ASA provocation challenges ($P = .0001$). Both tests had similar specificity whereas the oral test showed higher sensitivity. In both, concomitant urine leukotriene $E_4$ increases were found with the highest levels in patients with extrabronchial symptoms, suggesting the possibility of participation of inflammatory cells outside the lungs. This was the first comprehensive study to compare the 2 ASA challenge studies.

15. Sanak M, Pierzchalska M, Bazan-Socha S, **Szczeklik A**. Enhanced expression of the leukotriene C4 synthase due to overactive transcription of the allelic variant associated with aspirin-intolerant asthma. Am J Respir Cell Biol 2000; 23:290–6.

AIA, a distinct clinical syndrome affecting approximately 10% of adult asthmatics, seems unusually dependent on cys-LT overproduction by pulmonary eosinophils. The gene coding for $LTC_4S$, the enzyme controlling cys-LT biosynthesis, exists as 2 common alleles distinguished by an A to C transversion at a site 444 nucleotides upstream of the translation start. Andrew led the team that tested the hypothesis that this single-nucleotide polymorphism affects binding of transcription factors and influences the transcription rate, predisposing to AIA. Gel shift assay studies revealed that the $(-444)C$ allele, conferring an activator protein-2 binding sequence, is an additional target for a transcription factor of histone H4 consensus. Introduction of the H4TF-2 decoy oligonucleotide into $LTC_4S$-positive, differentiated HL-60 cells, decreased accumulation of $LTC_4$ to 68%. Transfection of COS-7 with promoter construct increased expression of β-galactosidase reporter for the $(-444)C$ variant. The $(-444)C$ allelic frequency was significantly higher in AIA patients (n = 76) compared with matched ATA (n = 110) and healthy controls (n = 75). Patients with

AIA also up-regulated LTC$_4$S messenger RNA expression in peripheral blood eosinophils. An inhaled provocation test with lysine-aspirin led to an increase in urinary output of LTE$_4$, which reached statistical significance only in carriers of the (−444)C allele. Their results suggested that a transcription factor, present in dividing and bone marrow resident progenitors of eosinophils, triggers LTC$_4$S transcription in carriers of a common (−444)C allele due to binding with the histone H4 promoter element of the gene. Genetic predisposition to cys-LT pathway up-regulation, a hallmark of AIA was, therefore, related to overactive expression of the LTC$_4$S (−444)C allele in some patients with AIA.

16. **Szczeklik A**, Nizankowska E, Bochenek G, Nagraba K, Mejza F, Swierczynska M. Safety of a specific COX-2 inhibitor in aspirin-induced asthma. Clin Exp Allergy 2000;31:219–25.

In a subset of patients with asthma, aspirin and several other NSAIDs that inhibit COX-1 can induce asthmatic attacks. Andrew and coauthors tested the hypothesis that in AIA patients the attacks are triggered by inhibition of COX-1 but not COX-2. In 12 AIA patients (7 men and 5 women, average age 39 years), oral aspirin challenges precipitated symptoms of bronchial obstruction with a fall in FEV$_1$ greater than 20% and a rise in uLTE$_4$ excretion. In 5 patients, the stable metabolite of PGD$_2$, 9α11β-PGF$_2$, increased in urine samples. The patients then entered a double-blind, placebo-controlled, crossover study in which they received either placebo or rofecoxib in increasing doses 1.5 mg to 25 mg for 5 consecutive days, separated by a 1-week washout period. No patient receiving rofecoxib developed dyspnea or fall in FEV$_1$ greater than 20%; mean uLTE$_4$ and 9α11β-PGF$_2$ urinary levels, measured on each study day for 6 hours postdosing, remained unchanged. Two patients, receiving placebo, experienced moderate dyspnea without alterations in urinary metabolites excretion. At least 2 weeks after completion of the study, all patients received an open challenge with rofecoxib (25 mg), without any adverse effects. NSAIDs that inhibit COX-1, but not COX-2, trigger asthmatic attacks in patients with asthma and aspirin intolerance. Rofecoxib can be administered to the same asthmatics without any adverse effects.

17. Zembowicz A, Mastalerz L, Setkowicz M, Radziszewski W, **Szczeklik A**. Safety of cyclooxygenase 2 inhibitors and increased leukotriene synthesis in chronic idiopathic urticaria with sensitivity to non-steroidal anti-inflammatory drugs. Arch Dermatol 2003;139:157

Thirty-six patients with chronic idiopathic urticaria (CIU) underwent oral aspirin challenge tests (up to 500 mg)—randomized challenges with rofecoxib (up to 37.5 mg) and celecoxib (up to 300 mg). After completion of the trial, 7 patients received naproxen sodium (500 mg) as a positive control. Aspirin-induced urticaria in 18 patients. Rofecoxib or celecoxib did not elicit urticaria in any of the aspirin-sensitive urticaria patients. Patients with CIU had higher baseline urinary excretion of LTE$_4$ than healthy control subjects. Basal urinary levels of LTE$_4$ and serum mast cell tryptase were increased in aspirin-sensitive urticaria patients compared with aspirin-tolerant patients. Severity and duration of aspirin-induced urticaria showed a positive correlation with uLTE$_4$ excretion. Naproxen precipitated urticaria in 5 of 7 aspirin-sensitive urticaria patients and also was associated with increases in uLTE$_4$. The investigators concluded that COX-2 inhibitors do not induce urticaria in the same patients with CIU who are known to be sensitive to NSAIDs. After inhibition of COX-1 but not COX-2, sensitivity to NSAIDs, in CIU, is caused by overproduction of cys-LTs and mast cell activation.

18. Mastalerz L, Setkowicz M, Sanak M, **Szczeklik A**. Hypersensitivity to aspirin: common eicosanoid alterations in urticaria and asthma. J Allergy Clin Immunol 2004;113:771–5.

Seventy-four patients with CIU and a history of sensitivity to aspirin and NSAIDs underwent placebo-controlled oral aspirin challenge tests. Concentrations of uLTE$_4$ were measured by ELISA and plasma stable prostaglandin D$_2$ metabolite, 9$\alpha$11$\beta$-PGF$_2$ by gas chromatoghraphy-mass spectrometry (GC/MS). All measurements were performed at baseline and after aspirin challenges. Patients were genotyped for the LTC$_4$S promoter single nucleotide polymorphism.

In 30 of 74 patients, aspirin challenges initiated urticaria/angioedema. In these 30 patients, baseline uLTE$_4$ levels were higher than in nonresponders and the healthy control subjects and significantly increased further after the onset of cutaneous reactions. No such increase occurred in subjects with negative aspirin challenge. Baseline uLTE$_4$ levels correlated with severity of skin reactions. Plasma 9$\alpha$11$\beta$-PGF$_2$ levels rose significantly in both aspirin responders and nonresponders, although in the latter group the increase occurred later than in the former. In patients who reacted to aspirin, frequency of ($-$444)C allele of LTC$_4$S was significantly higher than in patients who did not react. CIU, in patients with aspirin sensitivity, is characterized by the same eicosanoid alterations that have been demonstrated in AIA.

19. Wos M, Sanak M, Soja J, Olechnowicz H, Busse WW, **Szczeklik A**. The presence of rhinovirus in lower airways of patients with bronchial asthma. Am J Respir Crit Care Med 2008;177:1082–9.

Immunohistochemistry and the indirect in situ reverse transcription–polymerase chain reaction (PCR) methods were used to detect the presence of human rhinovirus (HRV) in bronchial mucosal biopsies in patients with asthma and nonasthmatic control subjects. HRV was found by immunohistochemistry in 9 of 14 bronchial biopsies from subjects with asthma (64.3%) and 2 of 6 nonasthmatic control subjects (33.3%) ($P = .38$). With the more-sensitive indirect in situ reverse transcription–PCR method, HRV was found in the mucosal biopsies of 73% of patients with asthma and 22% of nonasthmatic control subjects ($P<.001$). All 7 AERD patients had HRV in their bronchial biopsies. Subjects positive for HRV had lower pulmonary function, higher numbers of blood eosinophils and leukocytes, and eosinophilic infiltration in bronchial mucosa. This study, although not specific for AERD patients, nevertheless places the putative stimulus, namely the continued presence of HRV antigens, in all AERD patients studied in this early pilot study, and suggests that other derangements in the management of bronchial inflammation must be specifically faulty in patients with AERD.

20. Jakiela B, Szczeklik W, Plutecka H, Sokolowska B, Mastalerz L, Sanak M, Bazan-Socha S, **Szczeklik A**, Musial J. Increased production of IL-5 and dominant Th2-type response in airways of Churg-Strauss syndrome patients. Rheumatology (Oxford) 2012 Jul 5. [Epub ahead of print]

This is Andrew's last article, e-published in July 2012, 5 months after his death in February 2012. Churg-Strauss syndrome (CSS) is a rare systemic vasculitis associated with eosinophilia and asthma. The investigators assessed the local immune response in airways of CSS patients with different activity of the disease. Concentrations of IL-5, CCL17, CCL22, and CCL26 (ELISA) together with cell expression of T-helper–related genes (real-time PCR array) were measured in BAL fluid sampled from 11 patients with active CSS, 11 patients with CSS in remission, and 9 control subjects with bronchial asthma. In active CSS, both BALF and blood eosinophil counts were increased ($P<.01$). BALF cells in active disease were characterized by an increased expression of $T_H2$ and regulatory-type transcripts: STAT6, STAT3, GATA3, IL-4, IL-5, and IL-10 compared with asthmatics and STAT5A, CCR4, FOXP3, IL-4, IL-5, and IL-10 compared with inactive CSS. There was a significant increase in BALF concentration of IL-5 and CCL26 in exacerbation of CSS. CCR4-active chemokines were detected more frequently in active disease. We found a strong positive correlation between clinical parameters of disease activity (Birmingham Vasculitis Activity Score [BVAS], eosinophilia) and expression of IL-4, IL-5, IL-10, and STAT5A. These results indicated that, compared with asthma alone, active CSS patients had a much stronger local $T_H2$ response in the airways. Airway cells may contribute to lung eosinophilia in CSS by producing IL-5 and eosinophil-active chemokines.

After reading the above snapshots of Andrew's 20 publications, we were struck by his genius, innovation, and ability to make timely observations at the frontier of this exciting field. In addition, Andrew was a major collaborative scientist. The number of colleagues and authors from his own institution and across the world is truly astounding. Andrew's publications and collaborations were so important to the field of NSAID hypersensitivity that we can unequivocally write that he was the major force for advancement of understanding and treatment of these conditions.

As amazing as Andrew's academic accomplishments were to science and medicine, he was also a Renaissance figure with other extraordinary talents: he was a painter, played piano, and was known as a writer and essayist. His fascination with questions about how medicine and art share common roots and pose common challenges was reflected in his 2 successful and well-read books: *Catharsis. On the Art of Medicine*, in 2005 and *Kore. On Sickness, the Sick and the Search for the Soul of Medicine*, in 2007, translated into English, French, German, Hungarian, Lithuanian, and Russian. His last essay, "Immortality: Promethean Dream of Medicine, in 2012" was issued just a few days after his sudden death. This brilliant and beloved physician scientist, painter, artist, musician, and writer will be greatly missed by his friends and colleagues all around the world.

# Classification of Reactions to Nonsteroidal Antiinflammatory Drugs

Marek L. Kowalski, MD, PhD[a],*, Donald D. Stevenson, MD[b]

## KEYWORDS

- Nonsteroidal antiinflammatory drugs • Aspirin • Hypersensitivity • Adverse effects
- Aspirin exacerbated respiratory disease (AERD)

## KEY POINTS

- Adverse reactions to aspirin or other NSAIDs may occur in up to 30% of drug taking patients.
- Hypersensitivity reactions occurring in small number of patients taking NSAIDs may be either non-immunological (cross-reactive) or allergic (IgE or T-cell mediated).
- Assignment of a patient reaction to one of the specific categories allows for the application of the most effective diagnostic procedures.
- Proper classifications of the reaction may allow for type-specific patient management.

## HISTORY OF NONSTEROIDAL ANTIINFLAMMATORY DRUGS

Nonsteroidal antiinflammatory drugs (NSAIDs), including aspirin, are among the most commonly used drugs in the world, with billions of tablets taken over the counter or sold as prescriptions every year.[1] The history of their development is fascinating and dates back to the nineteenth century. Antipyrine was synthesized by German chemist Ludwig Knorr in 1883 and sold as an oral antipyretic and analgesic. Although not known at the time, antipyrine inhibits cyclooxygenase (COX). Antipyrine was sold as an oral drug under the name of Phenazone, until cases of agranulocytosis led to its discontinuation by the manufacturer in the 1930s. However, it is currently in use as one component of an ear drop, along with a local anesthetic benzocaine.

Acetylsalicylic acid, the second NSAID, was synthesized in 1897 by Felix Hoffman, who bound salicylic acid, extracted from willow bark, with acetic acid. Hoffman's father treated his own rheumatism with salicyclic acid, which induced an adverse effect of abdominal pain. Hoffman's unrealized hope was to relieve his father of

Disclosures: None.
[a] Department of Immunology, Rheumatology and Allergy, Medical University of Łódź, Lodz, Poland, [b] Division of Allergy and Immunology, Scripps Clinic and the Scripps Research Institute, San Diego, CA, USA
* Corresponding author.
*E-mail address:* Marek.Kowalski@csk.umed.lodz.pl

Immunol Allergy Clin N Am 33 (2013) 135–145
http://dx.doi.org/10.1016/j.iac.2012.10.008     immunology.theclinics.com
0889-8561/13/$ – see front matter © 2013 Elsevier Inc. All rights reserved.

abdominal pain by changing the molecule and thus decreasing gastrotoxicity, previously assumed to be a direct toxic effect of salicylic acid. Two years later, the molecule was commercialized by the Bayer Company under the name "aspirin," but Felix Hoffman, an employee of the company, received no royalties or compensation for his efforts. At the same time, aspirin started an amazing world career as a painkiller, antiinflammatory compound, and antithrombosis drug.

In 1922, Widal and colleagues[2] conducted oral challenges with aspirin and antipyrine in a patient with all the characteristics of aspirin exacerbated respiratory disease (AERD). Both aspirin and antipyrine initiated asthma attacks and profuse rhinorrhea during oral drug challenges, whereas chloral hydrate of quinine, urotropin, and pyramidon did not initiate any reactions. The second nonaspirin NSAID is phenylbutazone, which was introduced in 1952. It was followed in the 1960s by indomethacin and ibuprofen.[3] Since then, numerous COX-1 inhibiting compounds, with similar antiinflammatory activity and wide therapeutic applications for pain and inflammatory disorders, were synthesized and commercialized. However, with success comes problems, and the clinical efficacy of aspirin and other NSAIDs has been accompanied by a variety of common side effects during both short- and long-term therapies. Thus, designing less toxic compounds has continued to be an insurmountable challenge for pharmacologists of the twentieth and the twenty-first centuries as it was for Ludwig Knorr and Felix Hoffman at the end of the nineteenth century.

In 1971, Sir John Vane published his breakthrough discovery of the mechanism of antiinflammatory activity of aspirin and other NSAIDs.[4] In his Nobel Prize–winning experiments, he used a bioassay to demonstrate that NSAIDs share common pharmacologic effects, namely, inhibition of prostaglandin synthesis. His discoveries led to an understanding of the molecular mechanism of the activity of NSAIDs, which derives from their ability to specifically inhibit COX, originally called prostaglandin G/H-synthase, which is responsible for the biosynthesis of all downstream prostanoids (prostaglandins, prostacyclin (PGI$_2$), and thromboxane) (**Fig. 1**).[5] It is imperative that

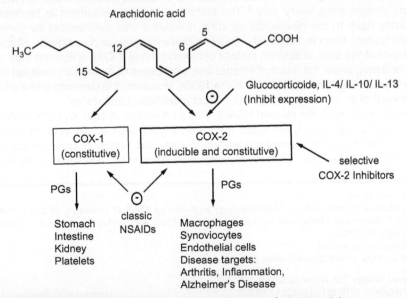

**Fig. 1.** Arachidonic acid metabolism and the mechanism of NSAID activity.

the allergy consultant understand this pharmacologic effect of NSAIDs because most of the positive and adverse effects of NSAIDs are through this pathway. COX, which is the first enzyme in the generation of prostanoids from arachidonic acid, exists in 2 distinct isoforms, referred to as COX-1 and COX-2.[6,7] COX-1 is expressed constitutively in most mammalian cells and is a major source of prostanoids that have important positive housekeeping functions, such as gastric epithelial cytoprotection by $PGI_2$. COX-2 is expressed either constitutively or after induction by inflammatory stimuli, hormones, and growth factors and generates prostanoids important for inflammation and is also involved in reproduction, renal physiology, bone resorption, and neurotransmission.[8] Discovery of COX isoforms prompted the development of molecules with selective inhibitory activity for COX-2, resulting in the introduction of a new class of NSAIDs, namely, COX-2 inhibitors (coxibs). These new compounds, although expressing strong antiinflammatory activity, have less gastrointestinal (GI) toxicity due to their preferential inhibition of COX-2 and inability to prevent the synthesis of COX-1 products, such as $PGI_2$, which is cytoprotective for gastric mucosa.[9] Both COX-1 and COX-2 inhibitors temporarily block COX enzyme channels and are therefore competitive inhibitors. Aspirin, on the other hand, acetylates COX enzymes, causing irreversible destruction. However, several reports have suggested that NSAIDs may also exert their therapeutic benefits by other mechanisms that are parallel to COX-1 inhibition (eg, direct inhibition of "inflammatory" transcription factors (nuclear factor-kappaB [NFkB]) or induction of resolvin generation). Thus, the understanding of their activities is still evolving.[10,11]

Differences in the molecular structures of NSAIDs may have important implications, not only for their shared ability to inhibit COX but also from an immunologic perspective. Their diverse molecular structures determine the differences in the capacity of specific NSAIDs to induce immune responses and the development of IgE-mediated or T-cell–mediated allergic reactions in susceptible individuals, which is the most confusing feature of reactions to NSAIDs. There is a group of molecules, with different structures, all of which block COX, with its confusing consequences. At the same time, each NSAID is uniquely antigenic, capable of sensitization in unlucky patients, followed by reexposure and a whole spectrum of immune reactions that are specific to that sensitizing NSAID. To make things even more complicated, some NSAIDs share epitopes and can therefore be recognized by antibodies or T cells, even though they are different NSAIDs (**Figs. 2** and **3**). Based on their similar molecular structures, NSAIDs have been categorized into several classes (**Table 1**), with some classes (eg, pyrazolones or oxicams) showing higher immunogenicity, leading to more frequent sensitization and anaphylactic reactions in sensitized patients.[12] Furthermore, structural similarities between NSAIDs tend to determine immunologic cross-reactivity, resulting in allergic reactions to drugs belonging to specific chemical classes.[13]

## ADVERSE REACTIONS TO NSAIDS

As with any drug, NSAIDs may be associated with the development of unwanted, adverse effects or reactions. According to the definition by the World Health Organization, an adverse drug reaction (ADR) is "a response to a drug that is noxious and unintended and occurs at doses normally used in man for the prophylaxis, diagnosis or therapy of disease, or for modification of physiologic function."[14] Thus, ADR is an umbrella description that covers any observed unwanted effects following the intake of the drug (regardless of the dose, timing, and host factors), providing there is a causal link between a drug and the observed undesirable effect (reaction). The most common adverse effects are in the digestive tract. Abdominal pain, occurring in 10% to 20% of subjects after a few days or weeks of ingesting daily NSAIDs, is the usual presenting

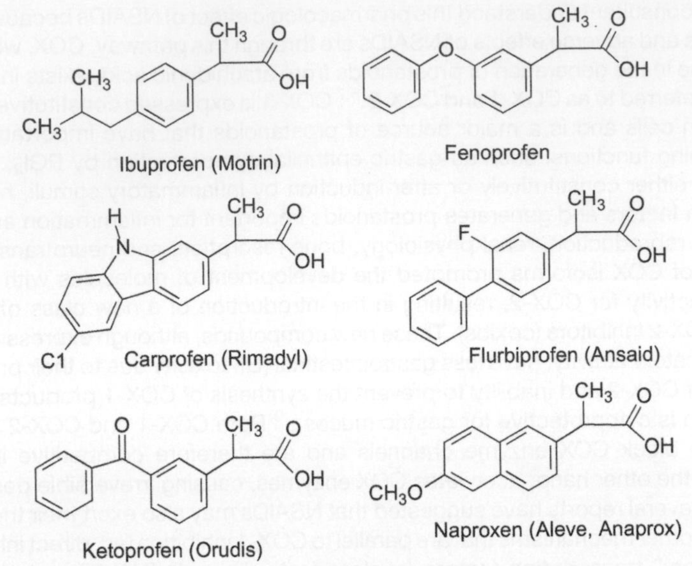

Fig. 2. Chemical structures of propionic acid NSAIDs.

symptom of NSAID-induced gastritis. It is due to the inhibition of COX-1 and the interruption of the synthesis of $PGI_2$. Likewise, increased bleeding, particularly in the skin, GI tract, genitourinary tract, and joints is a direct pharmacologic effect of aspirin through inhibition of thromboxane synthesis in platelets. It is rarely seen with the other NSAIDs.

However, in some patients, NSAIDs may induce acute adverse reactions in the skin (urticaria and angioedema, erythema multiforme, Stevens Johnson Syndrome [SJS], or toxic epidermal necrolysis [TEN]), respiratory tract (rhinitis, vocal cord spasm, or asthma attacks), or other organs (nephritis, hepatitis, pneumonitis, or anemia). Acute multiorgan systemic reactions such as anaphylaxis and chronic systemic reactions such as drug reactions with eosinophilia and systemic symptoms (DRESS) can also be caused by some NSAIDs.

From a practical standpoint, it is critical to distinguish between adverse effects occurring in otherwise normal patients (dose related) and NSAID reactions, which appear in small numbers of patients (non–dose related and possibly allergic). Although more recently pharmacologists proposed 6 categories of ADRs,[15] for the purpose of daily clinical practice a traditional classification distinguishing type A and type B ADRs might be more useful (Fig. 4).[16]

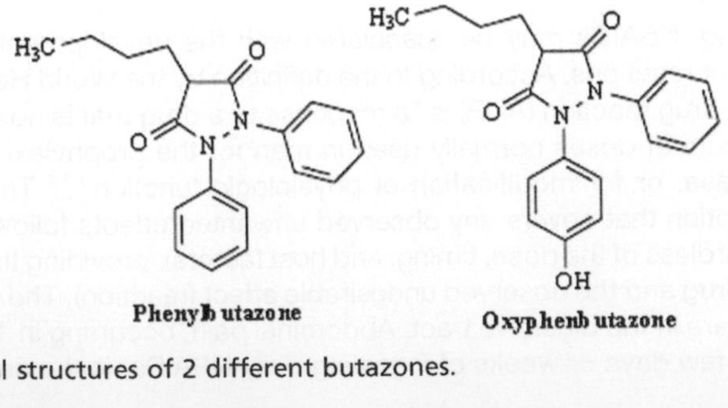

Fig. 3. Chemical structures of 2 different butazones.

**Table 1**
**NSAIDs grouped in classes determined by similar chemical structures**

| Group | Drugs |
|---|---|
| Salicylic acid derivates | Aspirin, sodium salicylate, choline magnesium trisalicylate, salsalate, diflunisal, salicylsalicylic acid, sulfalazine, olsalazine |
| Para-aminophenol derivates | Acetaminophen |
| Indol and indene acetic acids | Indomethacin, sulindac, etodolac |
| Heteroaryl acetic acid | Tolmetin, diclofenac, ketorolac |
| Arylpropionic acid | Ibuprofen, naproxen, flurbiprofen, ketoprofen, fenoprofen, oxaprozin |
| Anthranilic acid (fenamates) | Mefenamic acid, meclofenamic acid |
| Enolic acid | Oxicams (piroxicam, tenoxicam), pyrazolidinediones (phenylbutazone, oxyfentathrazone) |
| Alkalones | Nabumetone |
| Pyrazolic derivates | Antipyrine, aminopyrine, dipyrone |

*Data from* Sanchez-Borges M, Caballero-Fonseca F, Capriles-Hulett A, et al. Hypersensitivity reactions to non-steroidal anti-inflammatory drugs: an update. Pharmaceuticals 2010;3:10–8.

Type A reactions, also called dose-related or augmented reactions, are common and predictable, because they are related to the pharmacologic action of the drugs. They may occur in any healthy subject who takes a drug in sufficiently high doses. These reactions tend to have low morbidity and mortality and in some cases can be managed by dose reduction.

In contrast, type B reactions (called non–dose related or "bizzare") are less common, unpredictable, and associated with high mortality. Type B NSAID-induced reactions, which occur in a small fraction of susceptible patients and are of interest because they include various types of hypersensitivity reactions, are traditionally designated as allergic, pseudoallergic, or idiosyncratic. In agreement with the nomenclature recommended by the European Academy of Allergy and Clinical Immunology (EAACI)/World Allergy Organization, drug hypersensitivity reactions are defined as "objectively reproducible signs or symptoms initiated by a drug at a dose tolerated by

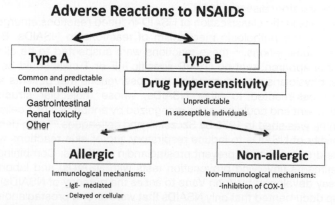

**Fig. 4.** Classification of NSAID-induced adverse reactions.

normal subjects" and are divided into immunologic (allergic) and nonimmunologic (nonallergic) reactions.[17,18] Thus, the term "drug allergy" should be used only for drug hypersensitivity reactions with a clearly defined immunologic (IgE- or non-IgE–mediated) mechanism, whereas "nonallergic" drug hypersensitivity should refer to other reactions with other pathogenic mechanisms. Accordingly, poorly defined terms traditionally used to described drug reactions, such as idiosyncrasy, pseudoallergy, or intolerance should be abandoned. This modern classification of drug hypersensitivity reactions has practical implications for diagnosis and management and can be directly applied to the classification of NSAID hypersensitivity reactions.[19]

## CLASSIFICATION OF NSAID-INDUCED HYPERSENSITIVITY REACTIONS

In 1902, only a few years after aspirin was commercially available, Dr Hirschberg from Poznań in western Poland reported the first case of a hypersensitivity reaction to aspirin manifesting as angioedema and dyspnea.[20] The first hypersensitivity reaction in an asthmatic patient was reported in 1910 by Dr Gilbert from Colorado,[21] and since then many different hypersensitivity reactions to aspirin affecting the skin, the respiratory tract, and other organs have been reported. The association of aspirin hypersensitivity, nasal polyposis, and asthma was described by Widal and colleagues[2] in 1922, and the syndrome defined as "aspirin triad" was characterized in a larger group of patients by Samter and Beers[22] in 1968. With the subsequent introduction of new NSAIDs, a variety of hypersensitivity reactions have been continuously reported.[23–26] The prevalence of NSAID hypersensitivity in the general population is high (varying from 0.5% to 5.7 %), and in some studies it is higher than allergy to antibiotics.[27,28] However, in high-risk populations, NSAIDs may induce hypersensitivity reactions in up to 20% in asthmatics with nasal polyps and pansinusitis (particularly in severe asthmatics) or 30% in patients with chronic idiopathic urticaria.[19]

Hypersensitivity reactions to NSAIDs vary in symptom (skin, respiratory tract, and solid organs), severity (from mild skin or respiratory reactions to severe generalized SJS/TEN or DRESS), and timing (may occur immediately after drug intake or weeks later). Over the years, the nomenclature of these reactions has become complicated and confusing because several poor descriptive terms have been used to describe various reactions (eg, aspirin allergy, idiosyncrasy, pseudoallergy, or intolerance), with little attention to the progress in understanding the mechanisms of these reactions. Samter and Beers[22] coined the term "aspirin triad" (nasal polyps, asthma, and aspirin-induced respiratory reactions). Triad has been replaced with the descriptor "aspirin exacerbated respiratory disease" (AERD).

Further progress in the classification of NSAID-induced reactions emerged with the understanding of the pathologic mechanism of reactions to NSAIDs. Before Max Samter's keen observations,[22] these reactions were suspected to be allergic. Over time, it became apparent that no NSAID-specific IgE or T cells could be identified. For decades, physicians were puzzled by the observations that patients sensitive to aspirin also cross-reacted to other NSAIDs, whose molecular structures were completely different and could never be recognized by antibodies or T cells. New light on that dilemma was shed in 1975 by Szczeklik and colleagues,[29] who demonstrated that the capacity of NSAIDs to induce respiratory and/or skin reactions was closely related to the drug's ability to prevent prostaglandin synthesis. Combining results of clinical experiments (involving provocation tests with NSAIDs) and laboratory tests (using bioassay developed by John Vane to asses the potency of NSAIDs), Szczeklik and his group documented that only NSAIDs that were strong prostaglandin inhibitors in vitro were capable of eliciting adverse respiratory reactions during clinical challenges In a subpopulation of asthmatics who are now known to have had AERD.[30] These experiments gave rise to the "prostaglandin hypothesis," which, for the first time, explained the phenomenon of cross-reactivity to NSAIDs observed in patients with asthma or urticaria. It was discovered later that NSAIDs block COX-1 and COX-2 but that only NSAIDs that are strong COX-1 inhibitors are capable of inducing adverse respiratory or skin reactions. On the other hand, selective COX-2 inhibitors are generally well tolerated, because COX-1 continues to function. This finding led to the follow-up "cyclooxygenase hypothesis."[31] According to this theory, in suscep-tible individuals, inhibition of COX-1, but not COX-2, by any NSAID, leads to an acute deficiency of protective prostaglandins, which in turn results in the activation of inflam-matory cells, with subsequent generation of potent mediators responsible for the development of symptoms of hypersensitivity. Originally, such a nonimmunologic mechanism was documented only for respiratory reactions occurring in patients with asthma/rhinosinusitis/nasal polyps, but it is now known that this also occurs in patients with chronic urticaria. To further complicate the picture, in some patients hypersensitivity reactions can be evoked only by a single NSAID or only a group of closely chemically related compounds (see **Figs. 2** and **3**), whereas other NSAIDs, with different chemical structures, are well tolerated.[32] In these patients developing either acute or delayed reactions, immunologic mechanisms of hypersensitivity are highly likely to be mediated by specific IgE antibodies or T cells.[33]

In 2001, Stevenson and colleagues[34] proposed a new classification of hypersensi-tivity reactions to NSAIDs, which was based on the spectrum of observed symptoms and included the presence or absence, in the affected patient, of the underlying chronic diseases (**Table 2**). Furthermore, for the first time, subtypes of hypersensitivity were defined while taking into account not only clinical descriptions but also putative pathologic mechanisms. This classification has been widely accepted and with minor modifications recommended for the diagnosis and management of patients with NSAID hypersensitivity.[19]

| Table 2 | | | |
| --- | --- | --- | --- |
| Classification of acute allergic and pseudoallergic reactions to NSAIDs | | | |
| Description of Reactions | Underlying Disease | Cross-reactions | Current Terminology |
| NSAID-induced rhinitis and asthma | Asthma/nasal polyps/sinusitis | Yes | Intolerance, ASA-induced, sensitivity |
| NSAID-induced urticaria/angioedema | Chronic idiopathic urticaria | Yes | Acute/chronic urticaria angioedema |
| Single drug-induced urticaria/angioedema | None | No | Acute urticaria/ angioedema |
| Multiple drug-induced urticaria/angioedema | None | Yes | Acute urticaria |
| Single drug-induced anaphylaxis | None | No | Anaphylactoid |
| Single drug- or NSAID-induced blended reactions | Asthma, rhinitis, urticaria or none | No or yes | Asthma and urticaria |

*Abbreviation:* ASA, acetylsalicylic acid.
*Data from* Stevenson DD, Sanchez-Borges M, Szczeklik A. Classification of allergic and pseudoal-lergic reactions to drugs that inhibit cyclooxygenase enzymes. Ann Allergy Asthma Immunol 2001;87:177–80.

## DEFINITIONS OF NSAID-INDUCED HYPERSENSITIVITY REACTIONS

Based on the original classification of Stevenson and colleagues,[34] further work has progressed and a new unified definitions of NSAID-induced hypersensitivity reactions have been proposed.[19] Five major distinct types of reactions have been identified, 4 acute, occurring within minutes to several hours after exposure and 1 delayed, developing more than 24 hours after exposure. It should be emphasized that other blended reactions that cannot be assigned into any classification are encountered in clinical practice.

### Aspirin Exacerbated Respiratory Disease

Hypersensitivity reactions, manifested primarily as bronchial obstruction, dyspnea, vocal cord spasm, ocular injection, and nasal congestion/rhinorrhea, occur in patients with underlying chronic airway respiratory disease (asthma/rhinosinusitis/nasal polyps). These patients have been said to have Widal syndrome, aspirin triad, asthma triad, Samter syndrome, aspirin-induced asthma or aspirin-sensitive rhinosinusitis/asthma syndrome, and aspirin-intolerant asthma. They are now called AERD.

### Aspirin Exacerbated Cutaneous Disease

Reactions manifested by urticaria and/or angioedema occur in patients with histories of chronic idiopathic spontaneous urticaria. This type of reaction was previously referred to as aspirin-induced urticaria or chronic idiopathic urticaria with aspirin exacerbation.

### Multiple NSAID-Induced Urticaria/Angioedema

Cutaneous reactions of urticaria and/or angioedema occur in otherwise healthy subjects who do not have a history of chronic spontaneous urticaria. At least 2 NSAIDs must induce urticaria, and these NSAIDs must have different chemical structures (do not belong to the same chemical group; see **Table 1**). This condition was previously called aspirin-induced urticaria.

### Single NSAID-Induced Acute Reactions

In this condition, wheals, angioedema, and/or anaphylaxis is evoked by a single NSAID or by 2 or more NSAIDs (belonging to the same chemical group). Other chemically non-related NSAIDs are well tolerated, and if these patients have a history of chronic urticaria it is coincidental. Previously used names are single drug-induced reactions and NSAID allergic reactions.

### NSAID-Induced Delayed Reactions

This condition is characterized by reactions to a single NSAID, developing within 24 to 48 hours to weeks after drug administration, manifested by skin reactions (eg, exanthema, fixed drug eruption), other organ-specific symptoms (eg, renal, pulmonary), or severe bullous cutaneous reactions.

## A STEPWISE APPROACH TO THE DIAGNOSIS OF A PATIENT WITH HYPERSENSITIVITY TO NSAIDS

Taking into account the diversity of mechanisms, proper assignment of a patient with symptoms of NSAIDs hypersensitivity to one of the aforementioned types of reaction is important because it includes the application of the most effective diagnostic procedures (provocation, skin testing, and/or in vitro testing) and may result in type-specific patient management. Patients want to know which NSAIDs to avoid and which can be used in the future. In addition to avoidance, recommending alternative NSAIDs or

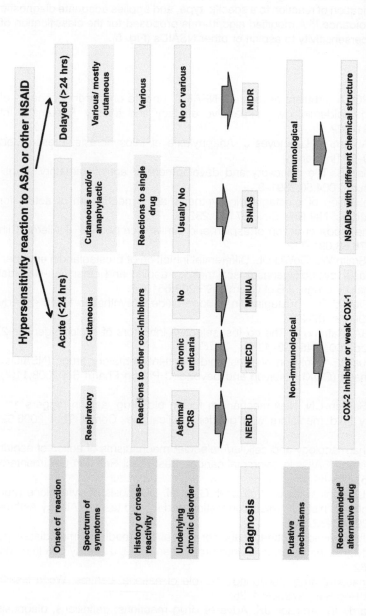

**Fig. 5.** Diagnosis and management of hypersensitivity to NSAIDs—a stepwise approach. AECD, aspirin exacerbated cutaneous disease; AERD, aspirin exacerbated respiratory disease; MNIUA, multiple NSAID-induced urticaria/angioedema; NIDR, NSAID-induced delayed reactions; SNIAR, single NSAID-induced acute reactions. [a] A tolerance test should be performed before the drug is recommended for regular use. (*Data from* Kowalski ML, Makowska JS, Blanca M, et al. Hypersensitivity to nonsteroidal anti-inflammatory drugs (NSAIDs) - classification, diagnosis and management: review of the EAACI/ENDA and GA2LEN/HANNA. Allergy 2011;66:818–29.)

other drug solutions is an important part of such allergy consultations. Furthermore, some drugs are innocent bystanders, and avoidance of drugs that have not caused reactions and have present or potential therapeutic benefits is not helpful and may even deprive the patient of a life-saving medication. EAACI Task Force on NSAID hypersensitivity proposed a diagnostic algorithm, which uses a stepwise approach, facilitates classification of reaction to a specific type, and applies adequate diagnostic methods and avoidance.[19] A modified algorithm is proposed for the classification of patients with hypersensitivity to aspirin or other NSAIDs (**Fig. 5**).

## REFERENCES

1. Conaghan PG. A turbulent decade for NSAIDs: update on current concepts of classification, epidemiology, comparative efficacy and toxicity. Rheumatol Int 2012;32:1491–502.
2. Widal MF, Abrami P, Lenmoyes J. Anaphylaxie et idiosyncrasie. Presse Med 1922;30:189–93 [in French].
3. Brune K, Hinz B. The discovery and development of antiinflammatory drugs. Arthritis Rheum 2004;50:2391–9.
4. Vane JR. Inhibition of prostaglandin synthesis as a mechanism of action for aspirin-like drugs. Nat New Biol 1971;43:232–5.
5. Vane JR. The mode of action of aspirin and similar compounds. J Allergy Clin Immunol 1976;58:691–712.
6. Meade EA, Smith WL, DeWitt DL. Differential inhibition of prostaglandin endoperoxide synthase (cyclooxygenase) isozymes by aspirin and other non-steroidal anti-inflammatory drugs. J Biol Chem 1993;268:6610–4.
7. Smith WL, DeWitt DL. Prostaglandin endoperoxide H synthases-1 and -2. Adv Immunol 1996;62:167–215.
8. Fitzgerald GA, Patrono C. The coxibs, selective inhibitors of cyclooxygenase-2. N Engl J Med 2001;345:433–42.
9. Rao P, Knaus EE. Evolution of nonsteroidal anti-inflammatory drugs (NSAIDs): cyclooxygenase (COX) inhibition and beyond. J Pharm Pharm Sci 2008;11(2): 81s–110s.
10. Chiang N, Serhan CN. New mechanism for an old drug: aspirin triggers anti-inflammatory lipid mediators with gender implications. Compr Ther 2006;32: 150–7.
11. Schrör K. Pharmacology and cellular/molecular mechanisms of action of aspirin and non-aspirin NSAIDs in colorectal cancer. Best Pract Res Clin Gastroenterol 2011;25(4–5):473–84.
12. Kowalski ML, Bienkiewicz B, Woszczek G, et al. Diagnosis of pyrazolone drug sensitivity: clinical history versus skin testing and in vitro testing. Allergy Asthma Proc 1999;20:347–52.
13. Himly M, Jahn-Schmid B, Pittertschatscher K, et al. IgE-mediated immediate-type hypersensitivity to the pyrazolone drug propyphenazone. J Allergy Clin Immunol 2003;111:882–8.
14. WHO. International drug monitoring: the role of national centres. World Health Organ Tech Rep Ser 1972;498:1–25.
15. Ralph Edwards IR, Aronson JK. Adverse drug reactions: definitions, diagnosis and management. Lancet 2000;356:1255–9.
16. Rawlins MD, Thompson JW. Pathogenesis of adverse drug reactions. In: Davies DM, editor. Textbook of adverse drug reactions. Oxford (United Kingdom): Oxford University Press; 1977. p. 10.

17. Johansson SG, Hourihane JO, Bousquet J, et al. A revised nomenclature for allergy. An EAACI position statement from the EAACI nomenclature Task Force. Allergy 2001;56:813–24.
18. Johansson SG, Bieber T, Dahl R, et al. Revised nomenclature for allergy for global use: Report of the Nomenclature Review Committee of the World Allergy Organization, October 2003. J Allergy Clin Immunol 2004;113:832–6.
19. Kowalski ML, Makowska JS, Blanca M, et al. Hypersensitivity to nonsteroidal anti-inflammatory drugs (NSAIDs) - classification, diagnosis and management: review of the EAACI/ENDA and GA2LEN/HANNA. Allergy 2011;66:818–29.
20. Hirschberg. Mitheilung uber einen fall von Nebenwirkung des Aspirin. Deutsch Med Wschr 1902;416:1906 [in German].
21. Gilbert GB. Unusual idiosyncrasy to aspirin. JAMA 1911;56:1262.
22. Samter M, Beers RF. Intolerance to aspirin: clinical studies and consideration of its pathogenesis. Ann Intern Med 1968;68:875–83.
23. Vanselow NA, Smith JR. Bronchial asthma induced by indomethacin. Ann Intern Med 1967;66:568.
24. Bosso JV, Creighton D, Stevenson DD. Flurbiprofen (Ansaid) cross-sensitivity in an aspirin-sensitive asthmatic patient. Chest 1992;101:856–8.
25. Gniazdowska B, Ruëff F, Przybilla B. Delayed contact hypersensitivity to non-steroidal anti-inflammatory drugs. Contact Dermatitis 1999;40:63–5.
26. Doña I, Blanca-López N, Cornejo-García JA, et al. Characteristics of subjects experiencing hypersensitivity to non-steroidal anti-inflammatory drugs: patterns of response. Clin Exp Allergy 2011;41:86–95.
27. Hedman J, Kaprio J, Poussa T. Prevalence of asthma, aspirin intolerance, nasal polyposis and chronic obstructive pulmonary disease in a population-based study. Int J Epidemiol 1999;28:717–22.
28. Kowalski ML, Demoly P, Pichler WJ, et al. Hypersensitivity to drugs and biological agents. In: Pawankar R, Canonica W, Holgate ST, et al, editors. WAO White Book on Allergy. WAO; 2012. p. 57–61.
29. Szczeklik A, Gryglewski RJ, Czerniawska-Mysik G. Relationship of inhibition of prostaglandin biosynthesis by analgesics to asthma attacks in aspirin-sensitive patients. Br Med J 1975;1:67–9.
30. Szczeklik A. Aspirin-induced asthma: a tribute to John Vane as a source of inspiration. Pharmacol Rep 2010;62:526–9.
31. Szczeklik A. The cyclooxygenase theory of aspirin-induced asthma. Eur Respir J 1990;3:588–93.
32. Czerniawska-Mysik G, Szczeklik A. Idiosyncrasy to pyrazolone drugs. Allergy 1981;36(6):381–4.
33. Pichler WJ. Drug hypersensitivity reactions: classification and relationship to T-cell activation. In: Pichler WJ, editor. Switzerland: Karger Drug hypersensitivity; 2007. p. 168–89.
34. Stevenson DD, Sanchez-Borges M, Szczeklik A. Classification of allergic and pseudoallergic reactions to drugs that inhibit cyclooxygenase enzymes. Ann Allergy Asthma Immunol 2001;87:177–80.

# Aspirin-Exacerbated Respiratory Disease: Clinical Disease and Diagnosis

Grażyna Bochenek, MD, PhD*,
Ewa Niżankowska-Mogilnicka, MD, PhD, FCCP

## KEYWORDS

- Aspirin-exacerbated respiratory disease • Aspirin • Aspirin hypersensitivity
- Nonsteroidal anti-inflammatory drugs • Provocation test • Aspirin challenge

## KEY POINTS

- Aspirin-exacerbated respiratory disease (AERD) is a distinct clinical syndrome of intractable inflammation of both upper and lower airways, which is characterized by the presence of asthma, chronic eosinophilic rhinosinusitis, nasal polyps, and hypersensitivity reactions to aspirin and other nonsteroidal anti-inflammatory drugs (NSAIDs).
- Exposure to aspirin and other NSAIDs does not initiate the underlying inflammatory process but only exacerbates clinical manifestations of the disease.
- AERD develops according to a distinctive pattern, characterized by a sequence of symptoms: persistent rhinosinusitis, commonly with polyposis, followed by asthma, and then aspirin hypersensitivity.
- Asthma runs a protracted course despite avoidance of aspirin and other NSAIDs.
- Provocation tests with aspirin are the most reliable method to confirm the diagnosis of AERD.

## INTRODUCTION

Aspirin-exacerbated respiratory disease (AERD) is a distinct clinical syndrome affecting both upper and lower airways, characterized by the presence of asthma, chronic eosinophilic rhinosinusitis, nasal polyps, and hypersensitivity reactions to cyclooxygenase 1 (COX-1) inhibitors, including aspirin and other nonsteroidal anti-inflammatory drugs (NSAIDs). Exposure to these drugs does not initiate the underlying inflammatory process but only exacerbates clinical manifestations of the disease.

---

Funding sources: None.
Conflict of interest: None.
Department of Pulmonology, Jagiellonian University School of Medicine, Jagiellonian University Medical College, Skawińska 8, Krakow 31-066, Poland
* Corresponding author.
E-mail address: graboch@tlen.pl

In line with the current classification, AERD belongs to cross-reactive types of hypersensitivity reactions to NSAIDs.[1]

The association of aspirin sensitivity, asthma, and nasal polyposis was described for the first time in 1922 by Widal and colleagues.[2] This syndrome was widely popularized in the late 1960s when Samter and Beers[3,4] described its natural history, and since then it was named *Samter's triad* or *the aspirin triad* (nasal polyps, asthma, and aspirin hypersensitivity). A fourth characteristic, chronic hyperplastic eosinophilic rhinosinusitis, was never mentioned in the description of "triad," but actually makes it a "tetrad"[5] However, neither description is particularly useful, because linkage to the respiratory tract is not disclosed and the original description was not made by Samter in 1968 but rather by Widal in 1922. AERD is now the preferred descriptor in North America and is gaining worldwide acceptance.

## PREVALENCE

The prevalence of aspirin hypersensitivity differs with respect to populations studied, diagnostic methods used, and criteria for defining hypersensitivity reactions. It affects 0.6% to 1.9% of the general population.[6–8] The prevalence was found to range from 4.3% to 11% among adult patients with asthma assessed with questionnaires,[6,7,9] and was even higher (21%) when provocation tests were used in patients with asthma and nasal polyposis and chronic rhinosinusitis.[10] In patients with asthma, chronic rhinosinusitis, and nasal polyps, the prevalence of aspirin hypersensitivity confirmed through oral aspirin challenge was found to range from 30% to 40%.[11,12] AERD is rare in children with asthma (2–5%) and is almost never seen before puberty.[10] Women outnumbered men by a ratio of 2.3 to 1 in Europe,[13] and 1.3 to 1 in the United States.[14] Family history of aspirin hypersensitivity was found in 1% to 6% of cases.[13,14] No racial or ethnic predilection to AERD was identified. The disease seems to be underdiagnosed in the population with asthma, because many patients who are aware of the risk of adverse reactions deliberately avoid NSAIDs. However, patients who experience mild NSAID-induced reactions do not associate them with drug ingestion or do not know that NSAIDs may cause asthma attacks.

## NATURAL HISTORY

The first symptoms of AERD usually appear between the third and the fourth decade of life.[15] In 2 large cohorts comprising 500 and 300 patients with AERD, the average ages of onset of the disease were 29 and 34 years, respectively.[13,14]

AERD can develop in patients who already have rhinitis and/or asthma or in those who have never had any prior respiratory disease. The clinical presentation is similar worldwide.[13,14] The disease develops according to a distinctive pattern, characterized by a sequence of symptoms: persistent rhinosinusitis, commonly with polyposis, followed by asthma, and then aspirin hypersensitivity. The first clinical manifestation is usually rhinitis, which is related to a flu-like infection. It is characterized by a watery discharge from the nose, nasal blockage, sneezing, and loss of smell. Rhinitis is perennial, difficult to treat, and progresses into a chronic hyperplastic eosinophilic rhinosinusitis often with nasal polyposis. Asthma is usually diagnosed 2 to 3 years later. At about the same time, the first unexpected adverse clinical reaction to aspirin or other NSAIDs occurs in patients who previously tolerated these drugs well. Some patients may have a diverse sequence of symptoms and NSAID-induced respiratory reactions, which are crucial for diagnosing AERD. Despite avoidance of aspirin and other NSAIDs, asthma runs a protracted course.

## CLINICAL PRESENTATION

The typical adverse reaction to aspirin or other NSAIDs includes symptoms from upper and lower airways. The first symptoms appear within 30 to approximately 120 minutes after ingesting a full therapeutic dose of a causative drug. Bronchospasm of varying severity is usually accompanied by profuse rhinorrhea, nasal congestion, conjunctival irritation, ocular tearing, and, rarely, periorbital swelling. Some patients experience skin rash and erythema of head and neck. The reactions may differ in their severity, ranging from isolated rhinitis to life-threatening anaphylactoid reactions with hypotension and loss of consciousness.[13,14] Individual patients experience nausea, stomach pain, and retrosternal pain. Vocal cord spasm can also occur during the reactions.

Asthma may vary in the degree of its severity. Some patients have mild or moderate disease. Others have severe chronic asthma requiring systemic corticosteroid therapy, frequent emergency department visits, or hospitalization from exacerbations. In the European cohort of 500 patients with AERD, 51% were treated with inhaled and oral corticosteroids, and a further 30% with high doses of inhaled corticosteroids to control their symptoms.[13] In the last year preceding participation in the study, 24% received intravenous corticosteroids because of asthma exacerbations.[13] Of the 300 patients with AERD in the United States, 77% were taking systemic corticosteroids in some pattern of use, such as every day, every other day, or as short courses, for treatment of exacerbations that occurred during the year before enrollment into the study.[14] The results of the TENOR study (the Epidemiology and Natural History of Asthma: Outcomes and Treatment Regimens) revealed that patients with AERD demonstrated more-severe bronchial obstruction and were more likely to have had emergency department visits, unscheduled office visits, hospitalizations, and corticosteroid bursts in the previous 3 months because of asthma exacerbations compared with patients with severe asthma who tolerated aspirin well.[16] In the European ENFUMOSA study, aspirin hypersensitivity was associated with more-severe cases of asthma.[17] In another study from Poland, the presence of NSAID hypersensitivity was a significant risk factor for severe refractory asthma.[18] AERD was highly prevalent among patients with near-fatal asthma in Japan.[19] In the European AERD cohort, asthma was more poorly controlled in women, as evidenced by a significantly higher number of emergency interventions and hospital admissions for asthma exacerbations.[13]

Most patients experience severe nasal blockage, postnasal drip, and loss of smell. Chronic rhinitis progresses into chronic eosinophilic hyperplastic rhinosinusitis with nasal polyposis, which is especially aggressive, frequently fills all sinuses, and may even invade bone structures. In the European cohort, rhinitis was present in 82% and nasal polyps in 60% of this population.[13] In the American cohort, almost all patients (99%) had nasal polyps.[14] In the same group, abnormal sinus opacifications were seen on plain films or CT in 99% of patients.[14] However, this high percentage may by biased by the high incidence of people referred for aspirin desensitization in that center. In another study, patients with AERD had a significantly higher rate of nasal polyps (90% vs 26%) and higher CT scores (16.9 vs 6.2) compared with patients with asthma who tolerated aspirin.[20] Chronic eosinophilic hyperplastic rhinosinusitis predisposes to secondary sinus infections, which may occur 5 to 6 times per year.[14] Nasal polyps have a tendency to rapidly regrow, resulting in multiple polypectomies and sinus surgeries in many patients. An average number of these surgical interventions estimated in 2 large populations of patients with AERD ranged from 2.6 to 3.0 per patient.[13,14]

In most cases, ingestion of aspirin or other NSAIDs by patients with hypersensitivity provokes both upper and lower airway response. However, a small subset of individuals have isolated nasal symptoms.[21] The reactions restricted to the upper respiratory tract during oral aspirin challenge were usually found in a mild and short-lasting disease.[22]

AERD is usually accompanied by increased eosinophil counts in blood, induced sputum, and nasal lavage.[15,23] However, particularly but not exclusively in patients treated with systemic corticosteroids, numbers of these cell counts can be within normal limits.

AERD can develop in patients who have both allergic and nonallergic rhinitis and asthma. The presence of atopy, determined by a skin prick test showing positive results to at least one aeroallergen, was found in 44% of this population.[24] In the same study, analysis of other definitions of atopy, including a combination of skin prick tests and history of atopy, specific and total IgE levels revealed that atopy was always more frequent in patients with AERD than in a general population without hypersensitivity to NSAIDs.[24] In a group of 103 German and Polish patients with AERD, positive skin prick test reactions to at least one aeroallergen were reported in 34%, increased levels of specific serum IgE (class $\geq 2$) against common allergens in 34%, and total serum IgE levels greater than 100 IU/mL in 46%.[13] Similarly, greater proportions of positive skin prick test reactions were found in the American cohort of 300 patients with AERD (66%), and in the TENOR study (92%).[14,16]

## RESPIRATORY REACTIONS TO ASPIRIN AND OTHER NSAIDS
### Strong COX-1 Inhibitors

Patients with AERD typically experience cross-reactions to aspirin and NSAIDs that are strong COX-1 inhibitors with a predominant preferential activity against this enzyme (Table 1).[25,26] The most common implicated analgesic both in Europe and the United States was aspirin, which elicited typical respiratory reactions in 80% of susceptible subjects.[13,14] Ibuprofen (41%), naproxen (4%), and ketorolac (1%) were the next most common NSAIDs to induce respiratory reactions.[14]

### Weak COX-1 Inhibitors

When given at a low dose (below 500 mg), acetaminophen (paracetamol), which is a weak COX-1 inhibitor, is safe in patients with AERD (Table 2). However, higher doses of this drug ($\geq 1000$ mg) elicit mild, easily reversed asthmatic reactions in some of these patients.[27] One study found that 34% of aspirin-sensitive patients with asthma reacted to acetaminophen in doses of 1000 to 1500 mg.[27] However, a recent meta-analysis revealed that only fewer than 2% of patients with asthma are likely to react to both acetaminophen and aspirin.[10]

### Partially Selective COX-2 Inhibitors

Meloxicam and nimesulide are preferential COX-2 inhibitors, and are usually well tolerated by patients with AERD when given at lower doses (Table 3). However, they can elicit respiratory reactions at higher therapeutic doses, because these doses can also inhibit COX-1. These reactions appear in a minority of patients and tend to be mild.[28–31]

### Selective COX-2 Inhibitors

Rofecoxib, celecoxib, and the less popular valdecoxib, etoricoxib, parecoxib, and lumiracoxib—all called coxibs—are highly selective COX-2 inhibitors (Table 4). They are the most recent class of NSAIDs and are well tolerated by patients with AERD. Rofecoxib and valdecoxib, however, have been withdrawn from the market because of increased incidence of cardiovascular side effects. Celecoxib is the only remaining

Table 1
Strong COX-1 inhibitors[a,b]

| Generic Name | Brand Name |
|---|---|
| Acetylsalicylic acid | Aspirin |
| Benoxaprofen | Oraflex |
| Diclofenac | Cataflam, Voltaren |
| Diflunisal | Dolobid |
| Etodolac | Lodine |
| Fenoprofen | Nalfon |
| Flurbiprofen | Ansaid |
| Ibuprofen | Advil, Motrin, Rufen |
| Indomethacin | Indocin |
| Ketoprofen | Orudis, Oruvail |
| Ketorolac | Toradol |
| Meclofenamate | Meclomen |
| Mefenamic acid | Ponstel |
| Metamizole | Pyralginum |
| Nabumetone | Relafen |
| Naproxen | Aleve, Anaprox, Naprosyn |
| Oxaprozin | Daypro |
| Piroxicam | Feldene |
| Tolmetin | Tolectin |

[a] Cross-reactivity between these NSAIDs is expected.
[b] COX-2 inhibition only occurs at higher doses.

selective COX-2 inhibitor available in the United States. Outside the United States celecoxib, etoricoxib, parecoxib, and lumiracoxib are available. Many well-designed, placebo-controlled studies revealed that this group of drugs does not cross-react with aspirin and other COX-1 inhibitors when taken in therapeutic doses by patients with AERD. These results were obtained during oral challenges with rofecoxib,[32–35] celecoxib,[36–38] and the remaining coxibs.[39,40] The results of these studies confirmed the hypothesis that inhibition of COX-1 is a critical event that triggers asthmatic attacks in patients with AERD. However, in some patients, hypersensitivity reactions to selective individual COX-2 inhibitors may occur.[31,41,42] The responsible mechanisms are not understood. For these cases, IgE-mediated reactions are likely,[43,44] and therefore the first full dose of a COX-2 inhibitor should be given to patients with AERD in a physician's office.

Table 2
Weak COX-1 inhibitors[a,b]

| Generic Name | Brand Name |
|---|---|
| Acetaminophen (paracetamol) | Tylenol |
| Salsalate | Disalcid |
| Azapropazone | Apazone |
| Choline magnesium trisalicylate | Trilisate |

[a] Usually well tolerated in AERD.
[b] Minimal COX-1 inhibition, without COX-2 inhibition at higher doses.

| Table 3 Partially selective COX-2 inhibitors[a] | |
| --- | --- |
| Generic Name | Brand Name |
| Meloxicam | Mobic |
| Nimesulide | Aulin, Nimesil |

[a] Preferential COX-2 inhibition at lower doses but partial COX-1 inhibition at higher doses.

## DIAGNOSIS
### Accuracy of the History

History of asthma attacks and nasal reactions after ingestion of COX-1 inhibitors and typical clinical presentation are highly suggestive. However, exclusive reliance on a history is not advisable. A multicenter European study showed that 15% of patients were unaware of their NSAID hypersensitivity,[13] and became informed of this diagnosis only after provocation tests with aspirin were performed. The indications that prompted physicians to perform these tests were the presence of asthma, nasal polyps, and/or sinusitis in patients avoiding aspirin and other NSAIDs. In one study 16% of consecutive patients with asthma and a prior history of NSAID hypersensitivity did not experience a reaction to aspirin during oral aspirin challenge.[45] Prior respiratory reactions could predict with some accuracy whether a positive oral provocation test result would occur, which also establishes the diagnosis of AERD. One study showed that patients with severe asthma attacks after ingestion of COX-1 inhibitors had a 100% chance of a positive result from an oral provocation test with aspirin.[46] Patients with a history of taking a NSAID and then having a mild or moderate prior asthma attack only once had a 73% to 79% chance of having AERD.[46] This chance increased to 89% when prior historical NSAID reactions occurred at least twice.[46] However, patients with nasal polyps, chronic rhinosinusitis, and asthma who were avoiding aspirin and other NSAIDs experienced positive results on oral aspirin challenges only 43% of the time.[46]

Thus, AERD could be both underdiagnosed or overdiagnosed when relying exclusively on a history of associations between asthma attacks and ingestion of NSAIDs.

### Provocation Tests with Aspirin

Provocation tests with aspirin are the most reliable method to confirm the diagnosis of AERD. No specific in vitro test exists. The following types of provocation tests exist,

| Table 4 Selective COX-2 inhibitors[a] | |
| --- | --- |
| Generic Name | Brand Name |
| Celecoxib[b] | Celebrex |
| Etoricoxib[c] | Arcoxia |
| Lumiracoxib[c] | Prexige |
| Parecoxib[c] | Dynastat |
| Rofecoxib[d] | Vioxx |
| Valdecoxib[d] | Bextra |

[a] Preferential COX-2 inhibition at prescribed doses, without COX-1 inhibition.
[b] Available worldwide.
[c] Available outside the United States.
[d] Removed from the world market in 2004 and 2005.

depending on a route of aspirin administration: oral, inhalation (bronchial), and nasal. In Japan and Korea, intravenous tests with aspirin are performed.[47] The principle of all tests is to deliver increasing doses (concentrations) of acetylsalicylic acid, followed by measurement of bronchial, nasal, ocular, and sometimes gastrointestinal or cutaneous reactions. Some patients react with a flush of their upper thorax. Associated urticaria, angioedema, vocal cord spasm, and hypotension also occur with less frequency.

Oral, inhalation, and nasal aspirin provocation tests do not differ significantly in sensitivity (89%–90%, 77%–90%, and 80%–86%, respectively) or specificity (93%, 93%, and 92.5–97.5, respectively).[48–51] However, a negative predictive value is higher for oral tests than for inhalation challenges (77% vs 64%).[48,49] Irrespective of the type of aspirin provocation tests used, they are performed based on 3 general indications:

- Suspicion of aspirin hypersensitivity based on a history of typical respiratory symptoms after ingestion of 1 or more COX-1 inhibitors.
- Suspected clinical presentation of AERD (eg, asthma, severe rhinosinusitis, and/or nasal polyposis) despite the lack of a clear history of prior NSAID reactions.
- As part of the aspirin desensitization process described in other articles elsewhere in this issue.

### Safety Requirements and Circumstances for Performing Provocation Test with Aspirin

Patients undergoing oral or inhalation tests with aspirin should be in a stable clinical condition and their baseline forced expiratory volume in the first second ($FEV_1$) should be at least 70% of the predicted value.[52] The tests must be performed in an outpatient or inpatient setting, under the direct supervision of experienced physicians, nurses, and skilled technicians. Emergency resuscitative equipment should be readily available. Nasal provocation tests are routinely performed in an outpatient clinic. It should be preceded by a rhinologic examination with anterior rhinoscopy to evaluate the presence of nasal polyps or any other abnormality that could interfere with the results of the test. Nasal inspiratory peak flow measurements can also be used and the equipment is not expensive.

In Europe, several asthma-controller drugs are temporarily discontinued before oral and inhalation tests (**Table 5**).[52] Oral and topical corticosteroids should be continued; however, the dose of oral corticosteroids should not exceed 10 mg/d of prednisolone or an equivalent because it may blunt the response to aspirin.[53] In the United States, patients are allowed to continue not only inhaled and oral corticosteroids but also long-acting bronchodilator. Leukotriene modifiers are routinely continued to prevent hyperirritability of the airways.[54] Only antihistamines, short acting $\beta_2$-agonists, and anticholinergics are discontinued for 24 hours before aspirin challenges.[54] Before

Table 5
Drug withdrawal before oral and inhalation provocation tests

| Drug | Time of Withdrawal |
| --- | --- |
| Short acting $\beta_2$ agonists | 6 h (8 h, if possible) |
| Ipratropium bromide | 6 h (8 h, if possible) |
| Long acting $\beta_2$-agonists | 24 h (48 h, if possible) |
| Long acting theophylline | 24 h (48 h, if possible) |
| Short-acting antihistamines | 3 d |
| Leukotriene modifiers | At least 1 wk |

nasal provocation tests, drugs that could blunt the response to aspirin should be also withdrawn (**Table 6**).[52]

### Oral Provocation Tests with Aspirin

Oral provocation tests with aspirin are regarded as the gold standard for diagnosing AERD. They are the most commonly performed, because the oral route mimics natural exposure and only a spirometer is required. Various protocols exist, which differ considerably in interval between administration of increasing doses of aspirin, total aspirin cumulative dose, and the criteria of the positivity of the test.

The oral provocation test worked up by the Task Force of HANNA (Hypersensitivity to Aspirin and other NSAIDs) together with the framework of GA2LEN Program, and accepted in Europe, takes 2 days.[52] On the first day, 3 capsules of placebo consisting of saccharine lactate are administered at 1.5-hour intervals. On the second day, aspirin with exponentially increasing doses are administered at 1.5-hour intervals until a cumulative dose of 500 mg is reached (**Fig. 1, Table 7**). $FEV_1$ is measured before each dose of aspirin and every 30 minutes thereafter. The test is interrupted if $FEV_1$ decreases 20% or more from baseline values (a positive reaction), or if the maximum cumulative dose of aspirin (500 mg or 1000 mg) is reached without a decrease in $FEV_1$ of 20% or more and in the absence of nasoocular symptoms (negative reaction). The results of the test could be also regarded as positive when unequivocal symptoms, such as severe nasal congestion, rhinorrhea, ocular injection, periorbital swelling, and erythema of skin and/or thorax, appear even if the $FEV_1$ does not decline by 20%. For positive results on provocative challenge test, the dose of aspirin causing a 20% decline of a baseline $FEV_1$ is calculated ($PD_{20}$).

In the United States only oral aspirin provocation tests are available (**Table 8**).[54] The oral challenge protocol lasts 2 or 3 days. The following reactions to aspirin can be distinguished:

1. Nasoocular symptoms alone
2. Nasoocular symptoms and a 15% or greater decline in $FEV_1$ (classic reaction)
3. Lower respiratory reaction only ($FEV_1$ declines by >20%)
4. Laryngospasm with or without any of the first 3 reactions
5. Systemic reactions: hives, flushing, gastric pain, hypotension

### Inhalation Provocation Test

Inhalation provocation tests are performed in several European centers.[48,49,52] They are not used in the United States because lysine-aspirin has not been approved for use in humans by the U.S. Food and Drug Administration.

| Table 6 | |
|---|---|
| **Drug withdrawal before nasal provocation tests** | |
| **Drug** | **Time of Withdrawal** |
| Nasal corticosteroids | 7 d (or the lowest possible dose kept through the aspirin challenge) |
| Oral corticosteroids | 7 d (or the lowest possible dose kept through the aspirin challenge) |
| Short acting antihistamines | 24 h |
| Nasal α-mimetics | 24 h |
| Oral α-mimetics | 24 h |
| Leukotriene modifiers | At least 1 wk |

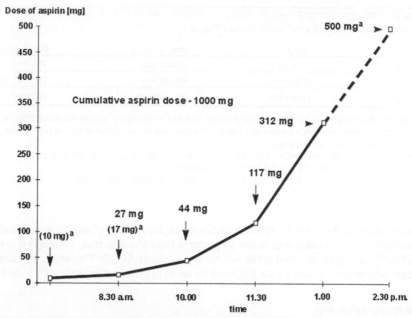

**Fig. 1.** Oral aspirin provocation test flowchart. [a] See **Table 7** for explanation. (*Data from* Niżankowska-Mogilnicka E, Bochenek G, Mastalerz L, et al. EAACI/GALEN guideline: aspirin provocation tests for diagnosis of aspirin hypersensitivity. Allergy 2007;62:1111–8.)

For inhalation provocation tests, which last 1 day, increasing doses of lysine-aspirin solution (a soluble synthetic analog of aspirin) are administered through a dosimeter every 30 minutes, and $FEV_1$ is measured every 10 minutes (**Fig. 2**).[52] The test is interrupted when $FEV_1$ decreases 20% or more from the baseline value or if strong extrabronchial symptoms occur (positive reaction). If the maximum cumulative dose of lysine-aspirin (218 mg) is reached without any adverse symptoms, the results are

**Table 7**
**The consecutive and cumulative doses of aspirin used in the oral provocation test (in Europe)**

| Consecutive Doses of Aspirin (mg) | Cumulative Doses of Aspirin (mg) |
|---|---|
| 10[a] | 10 |
| 27 | 27 |
| 44 | 71 |
| 117 | 188 |
| 312 | 500 |
| 500[b] | 1000 |

[a] Optionally, if a patient has a history of a severe reaction (severe dyspnea and/or anaphylactic shock) the provocation test should be started with 10 mg; the next dose of 17 mg is administered 1.5 hours later (ie, the 27-mg dose is divided into 2 doses for safety reasons).
[b] Optionally, if a patient with a strong suspicion of aspirin hypersensitivity shows no reaction after the final dose of 312 mg of aspirin (cumulative dose 500 mg), the next dose 500 mg can be administered 1.5 hours later.
*Data from* Niżankowska-Mogilnicka E, Bochenek G, Mastalerz L, et al. EAACI/GALEN guideline: aspirin provocation tests for diagnosis of aspirin hypersensitivity. Allergy 2007;62:1111–8.

| Table 8 An oral provocation test used in the United States | | | |
|---|---|---|---|
| Time | Day 1[a] | Day 2 (or 1) | Day 3 (or 2) |
| 8:00 AM | Placebo | 20–40 mg | 100–160 mg |
| 11:00 AM | Placebo | 40–60 mg | 160–325 mg |
| 2:00 AM | Placebo | 60–100 mg | 325 mg[b] |

[a] A placebo challenge can be conducted a week before; in patients whose baseline $FEV_1$ is the same as the previous best value and who have not used any rescue inhaler in the past week, the 1 day with placebo can be skipped.
[b] Patients who have not reacted to 325 mg will not react to 650 mg; therefore, the test should be stopped after 325 mg and the results considered negative.
*Data from* Stevenson DD. Aspirin sensitivity and desensitization for asthma and sinusitis. Curr Allergy Asthma Rep 2009;9:155–63.

regarded as negative. In the case of a positive reaction, $PD_{20}$ of aspirin is calculated. The inhalation test is safer and faster to perform than the oral test, although it is less sensitive.[48] Its negative result does not totally exclude AERD. Therefore, in case of a suspicious history, it should be followed by an oral provocation test with aspirin.

### Nasal Provocation Test

Nasal provocation tests are indicated in patients who cannot undergo oral or inhalation tests because of bronchial obstruction and severe asthma and in patients with typical symptoms of NSAID hypersensitivity exclusively in the upper airways.

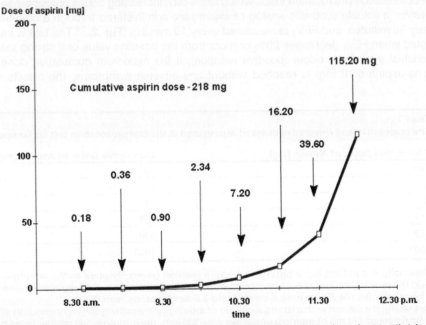

**Fig. 2.** Inhalation aspirin provocation test flowchart. (*Data from* Niżankowska-Mogilnicka E, Bochenek G, Mastalerz L, et al. EAACI/GALEN guideline: aspirin provocation tests for diagnosis of aspirin hypersensitivity. Allergy 2007;62:1111–8.)

Pulmonary function tests results are not a limitation for performance of nasal aspirin challenge tests.

After instillation of lysine-aspirin into the nostrils, the response is evaluated through recording nasal symptoms quantified with a visual analog scale and through using one of the following objective methods: acoustic rhinometry, active anterior rhinomanometry, or peak nasal inspiratory flow (PNIF).[50–52] A positive reaction is defined as the appearance of nasal symptoms, such as rhinorrhea, nasal congestion, sneezing, and a 25% decrease of total nasal flow compared with a baseline value measured with acoustic rhinometry or a 40% bilateral drop of inspiratory nasal flow compared with a baseline value measured with rhinomanometry or PNIFmeter. In the United States, the alternative to lysine-aspirin is challenge is a solution of ketorolac delivered as a nasal spray.[55]

The nasal provocation test is safe and rarely produces systemic reactions. However, a negative response does not rule out aspirin hypersensitivity and should be followed by oral aspirin provocation to make a definite diagnosis.

### Patient Supervision After Provocation Tests

Positive bronchial reactions are relieved through inhalation or nebulization of short-acting $\beta_2$-mimetics until $FEV_1$ returns within 90% of a baseline value. In the presence of more severe reactions, systemic corticosteroids are administered. Anaphylactic reactions require immediate intramuscular injections of epinephrine. Nasal obstruction is treated by topical $\alpha$-mimetics. In the presence of severe nasal symptoms, oral corticosteroids may be useful.

### Diagnosis In Vitro

Recently, the following in vitro tests were proposed to diagnose aspirin hypersensitivity in patients suspected of having AERD:

- Sulfidoleukotriene release assay, based on a potential capability of aspirin to induce $LTC_4$ release from peripheral blood leukocytes and, subsequently, on measurement of sulfidoleukotriene release.[56]
- Basophil activation test, in which expression of cell surface molecule CD34 is measured on in vitro challenge with aspirin.[57]
- 15- hydroxyeicosanoic acid (15-HETE) generation assay (ASPITest) is based on aspirin triggering generation of 15-HETE, an arachidonic acid metabolite, only in patients with AERD.[58]

Currently, none of these tests can be recommended for routine diagnosis of AERD, because their sensitivity and specificity have not been tested on large enough groups of patients, and results are inconsistent.[1,59]

### SUMMARY

AERD is a distinct clinical syndrome of intractable inflammation of both upper and lower airways, which is characterized by the presence of asthma, chronic eosinophilic rhinosinusitis, nasal polyps, and hypersensitivity reactions to aspirin and other NSAIDs. Exposure to aspirin and other NSAIDs does not initiate the underlying inflammatory process but only exacerbates clinical manifestations of the disease. AERD develops according to a distinctive pattern, characterized by a sequence of symptoms: persistent rhinosinusitis, commonly with polyposis, followed by asthma, and then aspirin hypersensitivity. Asthma runs a protracted course despite avoidance of aspirin and other NSAIDs. Provocation tests with aspirin are the most reliable method to confirm the diagnosis of AERD.

## REFERENCES

1. Kowalski M, Makowska JS, Blanca M, et al. Hypersensitivity to nonsteroidal anti-inflammatory drugs (NSAIDs) – classification, diagnosis and management: review of the EAACI/ENDA and GA2LEN/HANNA. Allergy 2011;66:818–29.
2. Widal MF, Abrami P, Lermoeyez J. Anaphylaxie et idiosyncrasie. Presse Med 1922;30:189–92.
3. Samter M, Beers RF. Concerning the nature of the intolerance to aspirin. J Allergy 1967;40:281–93.
4. Samter M, Beers R Jr. Intolerance to aspirin: clinical studies and consideration of its pathogenesis. Ann Intern Med 1968;68:975–83.
5. Lee RU, Stevenson DD. Aspirin-exacerbated respiratory disease: evaluation and management. Allergy Asthma Immunol Res 2011;3:3–10.
6. Kasper L, Sładek K, Duplaga M, et al. Prevalence of asthma with aspirin hyper-sensitivity in the adult population in Poland. Allergy 2003;58:1064–6.
7. Hedman J, Kaprio J, Poussa T, et al. Prevalence of asthma, aspirin intolerance, nasal polyps and chronic obstructive pulmonary disease in a population-based study. Int J Epidemiol 1999;28:717–22.
8. Gomes E, Cardoso MF, Praca F, et al. Self-reported drug allergy in a general adult Portuguese population. Clin Exp Allergy 2004;34:1597–601.
9. Vally H, Taylor M, Thompson PJ. The prevalence of aspirin intolerant asthma in Australian asthmatic patients. Thorax 2002;57:569–74.
10. Jenkins C, Costello J, Hodge L. Systematic review of prevalence of aspirin induced asthma and its implications for clinical practice. BMJ 2004;328:434–40.
11. Delaney JC. The diagnosis of aspirin idiosyncrasy by analgesic challenge. Clin Allergy 1976;6:177–81.
12. Weber RW, Hoffman M, Raine DA, et al. Incidence of bronchoconstriction due to aspirin, azo dyes, non-azo dyes, and preservatives in a population of perennial asthmatics. J Allergy Clin Immunol 1979;64:32–7.
13. Szczeklik A, Niżankowska E, Duplaga M, AIANE Investigators. Natural history of aspirin-induced asthma. Eur Respir J 2000;16:432–6.
14. Berges-Gimeno MP, Simon RA, Stevenson DD. The natural history and clinical characteristics of aspirin-exacerbated respiratory disease. Ann Allergy Asthma Immunol 2002;89:474–8.
15. Stevenson DD, Szczeklik A. Clinical and pathologic perspectives on aspirin sensitivity and asthma. J Allergy Clin Immunol 2006;118:773–86.
16. Mascia K, Haselkorn T, Deniz YM, et al, TENOR Study Group. Aspirin sensitivity and severity of asthma: evidence for irreversible airway obstruction in patients with severe or difficult-to treat asthma. J Allergy Clin Immunol 2005;116:970–5.
17. The ENFUMOSA Study Group. The ENFUMOSA cross-sectional European multi-centre study of the clinical phenotype of chronic severe asthma. Eur Respir J 2003;22:470–7.
18. Kowalski ML, Cieślak M, Perez-Novo CA, et al. Clinical and immunological deter-minants of severe/refractory asthma (SRA): association with Staphylococcal superantigen-specific IgE antibodies. Allergy 2011;66:32–8.
19. Yoshimine F, Hasegawa T, Suzuki E, et al. Contribution of aspirin-intolerant asthma to near fatal asthma based on a questionnaire survey in Niigata Prefec-ture, Japan. Respirology 2005;10:477–84.

20. Mascia K, Borish L, Patrie J, et al. Chronic hyperplastic eosinophilic sinusitis as a predictor of aspirin-exacerbated respiratory disease. Ann Allergy Asthma Immunol 2005;94:652–7.
21. Lumry WR, Curd JG, Zeiger RS, et al. Aspirin-sensitive rhinosinusitis: the clinical syndrome and effects of aspirin administration. J Allergy Clin Immunol 1983;7: 580–7.
22. Świerczyńska M, Niżankowska-Mogilnicka E, Zarychta J, et al. Nasal versus bronchial and nasal response to oral aspirin challenge: clinical and biochemical differences between patients with aspirin-induced asthma/rhinitis. J Allergy Clin Immunol 2003;112:995–1001.
23. Szczeklik A, Niżankowska-Mogilnicka E, Sanak M. Hypersensitivity to aspirin and non-steroidal antiinflammatory drugs. In: Adkinson NF Jr, Bochner BS, Busse WW, et al, editors. Middleton's allergy: principles and practice, Vol. 2, 7th edition. New York: Mosby Elsevier; 2009. p. 1227–43.
24. Bochenek G, Niżankowska E, Szczeklik A. Atopy trait in hypersensitivity to nonsteroidal anti-inflammatory drugs. Allergy 1996;51:16–23.
25. Szczeklik A, Gryglewski R, Czerniawska-Mysik G. Relationship inhibition of prostaglandin biosynthesis by analgesics to asthma attacks in aspirin-sensitive patients. Br Med J 1975;1:67–9.
26. Szczeklik A, Gryglewski R, Czerniawska-Mysik G. Clinical patterns of hypersensitivity to nonsteroidal anti-inflammatory drugs and their pathogenesis. J Allergy Clin Immunol 1977;60:276–84.
27. Settipane RA, Schrank PJ, Simon RA, et al. Prevalence of cross reactivity with acetaminophen in aspirin-sensitive asthmatic subjects. J Allergy Clin Immunol 1995;96:480–5.
28. Quarantino D, Romano A, Di Fonso M, et al. Tolerability of meloxicam in patients with histories of adverse reactions to nonsteroidal anti-inflammatory drugs. Ann Allergy Asthma Immunol 2000;84:613–7.
29. Bavbek S, Dursun AB, Dursun E, et al. Safety of meloxicam in aspirin-hypersensitive patients with asthma and/or nasal polyps. A challenge-proven study. Int Arch Allergy Immunol 2007;142:64–9.
30. Bavbek S, Celik G, Ediger D, et al. The use of nimesulide in patients with acetyl-salicylic acid and nonsteroidal anti-inflammatory drug intolerance. J Asthma 1999;36:657–63.
31. Bavbek S, Celik G, Ozer F, et al. Safety of selective COX-2 inhibitors in aspirin/ nonsteroidal anti-inflammatory drug-intolerant patients: comparison of nimesu-lide, meloxicam, and rofecoxib. J Asthma 2004;41:67–75.
32. Szczeklik A, Niżankowska E, Bochenek G, et al. Safety of a specific COX-2 inhib-itor in aspirin-induced asthma. Clin Exp Allergy 2001;31:219–25.
33. Stevenson DD, Simon RA. Lack of cross-reactivity between rofecoxib and aspirin-sensitive patients with asthma. J Allergy Clin Immunol 2001;108:47–51.
34. Martin-Garcia C, Hinojosa M, Berges P, et al. Safety of a cyclooxygenase-2 inhib-itor in patients with aspirin-sensitive asthma. Chest 2002;121:1812–7.
35. Woessner KM, Simon RA, Stevenson DD. Safety of high-dose rofecoxib in patients with aspirin-exacerbated respiratory disease. Ann Allergy Asthma Immunol 2004;93:339–44.
36. Woessner KM, Simon RA, Stevenson DD. The safety of celecoxib in patients with aspirin-sensitive asthma. Arthritis Rheum 2002;46:2201–6.
37. Gyllfors P, Bochenek G, Overholt J, et al. Biochemical and clinical evidence that aspirin-intolerant asthma subjects tolerate the cyclooxygenase 2-selective anal-getic drug celecoxib. J Allergy Clin Immunol 2003;111:1116–21.

38. Martin-Garcia C, Hinojosa M, Berges P, et al. Celecoxib, a highly selective COX-2 inhibitor, is safe in aspirin-induced asthma patients. J Investig Allergol Clin Immunol 2003;13:20–5.
39. El Miedany Y, Youssef S, Ahmed I, et al. Safety of etoricoxib, a specific cyclooxygenase-2 inhibitor, in asthmatic patients with aspirin-exacerbated respiratory disease. Ann Allergy Asthma Immunol 2006;97:105–9.
40. Valero A, Sanchez-Lopez J, Bartra J, et al. Safety of parecoxib in asthmatic patients with aspirin-exacerbated respiratory disease. Int Arch Allergy Immunol 2011;156:221–3.
41. Baldassare S, Schandene L, Choufani G, et al. Asthma attacks induced by low doses of celecoxib, aspirin, and acetaminophen. J Allergy Clin Immunol 2006;117:215–6.
42. Passero M. Cyclo-oxygenase-2 inhibitors in aspirin sensitive asthma. Chest 2003;123:2155–6.
43. Levy MB, Fink JN. Anaphylaxis to celecoxib. Ann Allergy Asthma Immunol 2001;87:72–3.
44. Stevenson DD. Anaphylactic and anaphylactoid reactions to aspirin and nonsteroidal anti-inflammatory drugs. Immunol Allergy Clin North Am 2001;21:745–68.
45. Pleskow WW, Stevenson DD, Mathison DA, et al. Aspirin-sensitive rhinosinusitis/asthma: spectrum of adverse reactions to aspirin. J Allergy Clin Immunol 1983;71:574–9.
46. Dursun AB, Woessner KA, Simon RA, et al. Predicting outcomes of oral aspirin challenges in patients with asthma, nasal polyps, and chronic sinusitis. Ann Allergy Asthma Immunol 2008;100:420–5.
47. Mita H, Higashi N, Taniguchi M, et al. Increase in urinary leukotriene $B_4$ glucuronide concentration in patients with aspirin-intolerant asthma after intravenous aspirin challenge. Clin Exp Allergy 2004;34:1262–9.
48. Niżankowska E, Bestyńska-Krypel A, Ćmiel A, et al. Oral and bronchial provocation tests with aspirin for diagnosis of aspirin-induced asthma. Eur Respir J 2000;15:863–9.
49. Dahlen B, Zetterstrom O. Comparison of bronchial and per oral provocation with aspirin in aspirin-sensitive asthmatics. Eur Respir J 1990;3:527–34.
50. Milewski M, Mastalerz L, Niżankowska E, et al. Nasal provocation test with lysine-aspirin for diagnosis of aspirin-sensitive asthma. J Allergy Clin Immunol 1998;101:581–6.
51. Alonso-Llamazares A, Martinez-Cocera C, Dominquez-Ortega J, et al. Nasal provocation test (NPT) with aspirin: a sensitive and safe method to diagnose aspirin-induced asthma (AIA). Allergy 2002;57:632–5.
52. Niżankowska-Mogilnicka E, Bochenek G, Mastalerz L, et al. EAACI/GALEN guideline: aspirin provocation tests for diagnosis of aspirin hypersensitivity. Allergy 2007;62:1111–8.
53. Niżankowska E, Szczeklik A. Glucocorticosteroids attenuate aspirin-precipitated adverse reactions in aspirin intolerant patients with asthma. Ann Allergy 1989;63:159–64.
54. Stevenson DD. Aspirin sensitivity and desensitization for asthma and sinusitis. Curr Allergy Asthma Rep 2009;9:155–63.
55. White A, Bigby TA, Stevenson DD. Intranasal ketorolac challenge for the diagnosis of aspirin exacerbated respiratory disease. Ann Allergy Asthma Immunol 2006;97:190–5.
56. Celik G, Bavbek S, Misirligil A, et al. Release of cysteinyl leukotrienes with aspirin stimulation and the effect of prostaglandin E2 in this release from peripheral

blood leukocytes in aspirin-induced asthmatic patients. Clin Exp Allergy 2001;31: 1615–22.

57. Gamboa P, Sanz ML, Caballero MR, et al. The flow-cytometric determination of basophil activation induced by aspirin and other non-steroidal anti-inflammatory drugs (NSAIDs) is useful for in vitro diagnosis of the NSAID hypersensitivity syndrome. Clin Exp Allergy 2004;34:1448–57.

58. Kowalski ML, Ptasińska A, Jędrzejczak M, et al. Aspirin-triggered 15-HETE generation in peripheral blood leukocytes is a specific and sensitive Aspirin-Sensitive Patients Identification Test (ASPITest). Allergy 2005;60:1139–45.

59. Ebo DG, Leysen J, Mayorga C, et al. The *in vitro* diagnosis of drug allergy: status and perspectives. Allergy 2001;66:1275–86.

# Rhinosinusitis and Nasal Polyps in Aspirin-Exacerbated Respiratory Disease

Joaquim Mullol, MD, PhD[a,b,c,d,*], César Picado, MD, PhD[b,c,d,e]

## KEYWORDS

- Aspirin • Aspirin desensitization • Aspirin-exacerbated respiratory disease (AERD)
- Chronic rhinosinusitis • Corticosteroids • Nasal polyps
- Nonsteroidal antiinflammatory drugs (NSAID)

## KEY POINTS

- Aspirin/nonsteroidal antiinflammatory drug sensitivity is common in patients with chronic rhinosinusitis (CRS) and nasal polyps, causing a more severe disease, referred to as aspirin-exacerbated respiratory disease (AERD).
- The nasal polyps and CRS, which are the cornerstone of the diagnosis of AERD, are generally difficult to treat.
- Medication, particularly intranasal spray or corticosteroids in drops, constitutes the first line of treatment of patients with CRS with nasal polyps and AERD.
- Endoscopic sinus surgery is recommended when medication fails, and a follow-up and medication, including nasal and oral corticosteroids, are recommended after surgery.
- Aspirin desensitization, followed by daily aspirin treatment, is presented elsewhere in this issue in the article on aspirin desensitization in AERD.

Funding support: The research group is sponsored in part by Generalitat de Catalunya, Centro de Investigaciones Biomédicas en Red de Enfermedades Respiratorias (CIBERES), and Global Allergy and Asthma European Network (GA²LEN eV).

Disclosure: Dr Mullol is or has been lecturer and/or member of National and/or International Scientific Advisory Boards for Boheringer-Ingelheim, Esteve, FAES, Grupo Uriach, GSK, Hartington Pharmaceuticals, Johnson & Johnson, MEDA, MSD, Novartis, Pierre-Fabre, and UCB Pharchim. He has received grants for research projects from FAES, Grupo Uriach, GSK, MSD, and UCB Pharchim; and has been national and/or international coordinator and/or main investigator of clinical trials for FAES, Grupo Uriach, GSK, MSD, Pierre-Fabre, and UCB Pharchim. Dr Picado is or has been lecturer and/or member of National and/or International Scientific Advisory Boards for FAES, Grupo Uriach, MSD, Novartis, and Stallergens. He has received grants for research projects from MSD, Novartis, Chiesi, Grupo Uriach, Leti, and Stallergens, and has been national and/or international coordinator and/or main investigator of clinical trials for AstraZeneka, GSK, Novartis and MSD.

[a] Rhinology Unit & Smell Clinic, Department of Otorhinolaryngology, Hospital Clínic i Universitari, University of Barcelona, c/Villarroel, 170, Barcelona 08036, Catalonia, Spain; [b] Clinical and Experimental Respiratory Immunoallergy, Institut d'Investigacions Biomèdiques August Pi i Sunyer (IDIBAPS), Barcelona, Catalonia, Spain; [c] Centro de Investigación Biomédica en Red de Enfermedades Respiratorias (CIBERES), Barcelona 08036, Catalonia, Spain; [d] Global Allergy and Asthma European Network (GA²LEN), Barcelona 08036, Catalonia, Spain; [e] Allergy Unit, Department of Pneumology and Respiratory Allergy, Hospital Clínic i Universitari, University of Barcelona, c/Villarroel, 170, Barcelona 08036, Catalonia, Spain
* Corresponding author.
E-mail address: jmullol@clinic.ub.es

Immunol Allergy Clin N Am 33 (2013) 163–176
http://dx.doi.org/10.1016/j.iac.2012.11.002
0889-8561/13/$ – see front matter © 2013 Elsevier Inc. All rights reserved.

## INTRODUCTION

The presence of aspirin-exacerbated respiratory disease (AERD) in a patient with chronic rhinosinusitis with nasal polyps (CRSwNP) and asthma is associated with severe eosinophilic upper and lower airway disease. This article deals with the inflammatory disease of the respiratory tract as it relates to the sinuses. Involvement of the sinuses in AERD is almost universal, depending on the stage of onset of the disease and evaluation by computed tomography (CT). A patient with normal sinus CT, asthma, and rhinitis, almost without exception, does not have a positive, oral, nasal, or inhalation aspirin challenge to aspirin and therefore does not have AERD. Thus, CRS is central to AERD. This article explores the clinical aspects, physiopathology, and treatment of rhinosinusitis as it relates to AERD.

## DEFINITIONS

### CRS

The diagnosis of CRS with or without NP is mainly based on clinical history (presence and duration for more than 12 weeks of sinonasal symptoms), nasal endoscopy, and CT scan of the paranasal sinuses.[1-4]

In the 2012 update of the EPOS international rhinosinusitis guidelines,[1,2] CRSwNP was defined as inflammation of the sinonasal mucosa with the presence of at least 2 sinonasal symptoms, one of these being nasal blockage/obstruction/congestion or nasal discharge (anterior rhinorrhea/posterior nasal drip), facial pain/pressure, or reduction or loss of smell for more than 12 weeks. Endoscopic signs of NP, edema/mucosal obstruction in the middle meatus, or CT changes within the ostiomeatal complex or paranasal sinuses help form a definitive diagnosis.

As recorded by CT, CRS in patients with AERD with nasal polyposis is characterized by the involvement of all paranasal sinuses and nasal passages and the thickness of hypertrophic mucosa in up to 100% of the patients, to a greater extent than in aspirin-tolerant patients.[5] Patients with AERD have significantly worse preoperative CT and nasal endoscopy scores than aspirin-tolerant patients.[6]

## EPIDEMIOLOGY AND NATURAL HISTORY

CRS, with or without NP, affects 11% and 14% of the European[7] and American[8] general populations, respectively. CRSwNP is an inflammatory condition of the nose and paranasal sinuses of unknown cause, which is present in 2% to 4% of the adult population.[1,2] CRSwNP is often associated with other respiratory diseases such as asthma,[9] aspirin sensitivity,[10] and idiopathic bronchiectasis.[11] The presence of hypersensitivity to aspirin or other nonsteroidal antiinflammatory drugs (NSAIDs) in a patient with CRSwNP[12,13] is usually associated with a particularly severe, persistent, and treatment-resistant form of the disease, usually coexisting with severe asthma.

AERD has been reported in 8% to 26% of patients with CRSwNP and in 10% to 20% of asthmatic patients.[14] The prevalence of nasal polyposis in aspirin-sensitive asthmatics may be as high as 60% to 70%, compared with less than 10% in the population of aspirin-tolerant asthmatics.[15] The precise prevalence of nasal polyposis in AERD is difficult to document, because tiny polyps in and around the middle meatus may be obscured by swollen turbinates, and nasal endoscopy needs to be performed. In addition, shrinkage of polyps after systemic corticosteroids may give a false-negative conclusion in such studies when examination is not repeated after regrowth of polyps. Thus, in AERD, the true prevalence may be closer to 100%. The increased severity of the upper airway disease in these patients is reflected by the high recurrence of NP and frequent need for endoscopic sinus surgery.[16]

Furthermore, CRS and nasal polyposis have an important impact on the patient's quality of life,[17] which is worsened by the presence of atopy[18] and asthma,[19] although there is a clear improvement after both medical and surgical treatments.[20] The socioeconomic burden of CRS and nasal polyposis is also considerable. In the United States, the direct treatment cost of CRS has been estimated at 3.4 to 5 US$ billion annually,[21] whereas the average surgical costs of functional endoscopic sinus surgery and postsurgical care have been calculated as 7726 US$ per patient.[22] In consequence, the health care cost is burdensome in patients with AERD, who receive 3 sinus operations on average.[23]

In the natural course of the syndrome, a clinical history of rhinitis or CRS usually precedes asthma and the development of aspirin hypersensitivity. In the AIANE (European Network on Aspirin-Induced Asthma) cohort study, the disease followed a typical pattern[10]: persistent rhinitis/rhinosinusitis appeared first (mean age 30 years), being related to a flulike infection in half of the patients; this was followed by asthma after 2 years, on average (mean age 32 years), and by aspirin-induced respiratory reactions and nasal polyposis after 4 years (mean age 34 years). The clinical presentation in the different European countries was remarkably similar. In women, who outnumbered men by a ratio of 2.3:1, the onset of symptoms occurred significantly earlier and the disease was more severe than in men. Once developed, RSC and asthma follow a course that is usually independent of the aspirin and NSAID avoidance.[23]

## PATHOPHYSIOLOGY
### Cells and Cytokines

CRSwNP is characterized by an intense inflammatory process with perivascular and subepithelial inflammatory cell infiltration, edematous stroma, and formation of pseudocysts. In most patients with CRSwNP, eosinophils are the predominant infiltrating cells.[24] The most intense eosinophilic infiltration is usually found in CRSwNP associated with AERD.[25]

However, recent studies suggest that the dominant inflammatory cell can vary according to the racial characteristics of the population. In contrast with the predominant eosinophilic infiltration detected in whites, neutrophils seem to dominate in Chinese patients with CRSwNP.[26] The mechanisms involved in this difference have yet to be clarified.

The recruitment of eosinophils is regulated by various cytokines and vascular adhesion molecules. Increased production of interleukin 5 (IL-5), eotaxins, and RANTES (regulated on activation, normal T-cell expressed, and secreted) has been reported in CRSwNP.[25,27–29] The highest production of cytokines involved in eosinophil recruitment and activation, such as IL-5, is found in the nasal tissue of patients with CRSwNP and AERD; this explains why these patients showed the most intense eosinophilic inflammatory process.[25] Moreover, increased expression of vascular adhesion molecule 1 (VCAM-1) has been detected in CRSwNP and correlated with the level of tissue eosinophilia, suggesting a role for VCAM-1 in eosinophil recruitment to the inflamed CRSwNP tissue.[30]

Activated lymphocyte, Th2 polarized infiltration is characteristic of CRSwNP as indicated by the predominance of cytokine signals, such as IL-5, a cytokine associated with the Th2 lymphocyte subset.[31]

Mast cells are also abundant in CRSwNP tissue, especially in those with associated AERD.[32] The number of mast cells was correlated with the number of polypectomies, suggesting that mast cell activity is involved in the pathogenesis of nasal polyposis.

### Arachidonic Acid Metabolism in CRSwNP with and Without AERD

Arachidonic acid (AA) is formed from the phospholipids of cell membranes by the action of phospholipase $A_2$. AA can be metabolized by various enzymes such as cyclooxygenase (Cox), and 5-lipoxygenase (5-LO).[33]

Cox is found in different isoforms known as Cox-1 and Cox-2. Cox-1 is generally constitutively expressed and considered a housekeeping gene,[33] whereas Cox-2 is induced under chronic inflammatory conditions.[34–36] Several prostaglandins (PGs) are synthesized as a result of Cox-2 activation; these are known as $PGE_2$, $PGF_{2\alpha}$, and $PGD_2$. $PGD_2$ and $PGF_{2\alpha}$ are bronchoconstrictors and $PGD_2$ is released by mast cells during allergic reactions.[33]

$PGE_2$ can perform contrasting activities, such as bronchodilation and bronchoconstriction in the airways, and antiinflammatory and proinflammatory actions in the lung.[37] The origin of the various $PGE_2$ actions seems to partly depend on the different types of cell surface receptors that may be stimulated by this PG. There are 4 different $PGE_2$ receptors: $EP_1$ to $EP_4$. The stimulation of $EP_2$ and $EP_4$ results in relaxing effects. In contrast, $EP_1$ acts as a constrictor, whereas $EP_3$ (various isoforms of which are known to result from a splicing process) is considered an inhibitor receptor. The presence or predominance of any given type of receptor in cells could explain the different effects induced by $PGE_2$.[38] The Cox-1 pathway is the target for classic NSAIDs, whereas coxibs are selective Cox-2 inhibitors.[39]

AA can also be metabolized through the 5-LO pathway. 5-LO is mostly found in cells that are involved in inflammatory responses, such as eosinophils, neutrophils, mast cells, and macrophages. 5-LO is usually located in the cytoplasm; it translocates toward the nuclear membrane to interact with its processing protein, called FLAP, thus enabling it to oxygenate the AA to form a hydroperoxide (5-HPETE), which in turn is converted into leukotriene $A_4$ ($LTA_4$) by the 5-LO. In some cells, $LTA_4$ can be transformed into $LTB_4$ by an $LTA_4$ hydrolase or into $LTC_4$ by an $LTC_4$ synthase enzyme (LT-$C_4$S). The $LTC_4$ is exported toward the exterior of the cells, where it is later metabolized into $LTD_4$ and $LTE_4$ by a $\gamma$-glutamyl-transpeptidase and a dipeptidase, respectively. $LTC_4$, $LTD_4$, and $LTE_4$ form the so-called cysteinyl leukotrienes (Cys-LTs), previously known as the slow-reacting substance of anaphylaxis. Cys-LTs are powerful bronchoconstrictors, which enhance edema formation and are chemotactic for eosinophils.[40]

Cys-LTs act as agonists to at least 2 receptors: Cys-$LT_1$ and Cys-$LT_2$. The former is widely distributed in inflammatory cells and seems to intervene in rhinitis and asthma reactions, whereas the latter is located predominantly in the blood vessels and its function is still unknown.[40]

AA can also be metabolized by a more complex mechanism called transcellular biosynthesis, whereby at least 2 different types of cells work together. The result of this combined activity is the synthesis of lipoxins (LXs) $LXA_4$, $LXB_4$, 15-epi-$LXA_4$, and 15-epi-$LXB_4$. Their synthesis occurs via 3 transcellular routes: the first involves the generation of $LTA_4$ by the 5-LO present in cells of myeloid lineage, which are taken up by platelets, where $LTA_4$ is metabolized by the enzyme 12-LO to form $LX_4$. A second route involves the generation of 15-hydroxyeicosatetraenoic acid (15 [S]-HETE) by 15-LO of epithelial or monocyte cells, which serves as a substrate for 5-LO in neutrophils to produce $LX_4$ and $LXB_4$. There is also a third route involving Cox-2 and 5-LO, in the so-called aspirin-triggered 15-epi-LX pathway. In this pathway, aspirin causes the blockage of the catalytic activity of Cox-2, which becomes unable to produce PGs. At the same time, the Cox-2 acquires the ability to produce 15(S)-HETE, which is converted by the 5-LO of leukocytes into epimers of LXs (15-epi-LXA$_4$ and 15-epi-LXB$_4$).

LXs have powerful antiinflammatory properties, including the inhibition of chemotaxis and the adherence and endothelial transmigration of neutrophils.

### AA metabolism in CRSwNP

**Cox pathway** Various studies have reported low PGE$_2$ production in CRSwNP of patients with and without aspirin intolerance, compared with control nasal mucosa.[25,41] The deficient production of PGE$_2$ was greater in aspirin-intolerant than in aspirin-tolerant patients.

Given the dependence of PGE$_2$ production on Cox-1 and Cox-2 activity, the expression of both enzymes has been assessed in nasal mucosa and in NP. Cox-1 is usually considered an enzyme that responds to the physiologic needs of cells but is not involved in inflammatory responses. However, some studies have shown mild increases in its expression in inflamed tissues.[33] A substantial upregulation of Cox-1 has been reported in CRSwNP associated with cystic fibrosis, a finding that suggests that airway Cox-1 is sensitive to inflammatory stimuli.[35] However, other studies on the regulation of Cox-1 in CRSwNP of patients with and without aspirin intolerance have yielded contradictory results. Some studies have reported no differences at baseline in Cox-1 expression between nasal mucosa and NP from either asthma-tolerant or asthma-intolerant asthmatics,[42,43] whereas others using proinflammatory stimulation have reported a lower Cox-1 expression in fibroblasts of NP derived from patients with asthma-intolerant asthma compared with healthy nasal mucosa.[41]

Because Cox-2 expression increases in inflammatory processes, a concomitant alteration in the expression of Cox-2 would be expected to complement the changes in PGE$_2$ levels detected in NP. In line with the results reported with PGE$_2$, Cox-2 expression has been shown to be downregulated in NP of patients with and without aspirin hypersensitivity[25,41–45] through a potential Nuclear Factor κ B–mediated downregulation.[46] However, other studies failed to find any difference in the expression of Cox-2 in the NP of aspirin-intolerant, aspirin-tolerant, and control individuals.[47]

There are no clear explanations to account for the discrepancies reported in the regulation of the 2 Cox enzymes in asthma and NP. Differences in the methods used in the identification and quantification of enzymes probably help explain these discrepancies. In general, the studies that used real-time polymerase chain reaction and Western blot techniques found low expression of the enzymes, whereas those using immunohistochemistry found contradictory results, with low or similar expression of Cox-2 in NP compared with nasal mucosa. It has been suggested that discrepancies may result from the use of polyclonal or monoclonal antibodies.[48] The accuracy of this methodology can also be limited in studies of tissues samples with different cell composition, such as healthy nasal mucosa and inflamed NP infiltrated by numerous inflammatory cells. To overcome these technical limitations, a recent study assessed Cox-2 expression, with enzyme-linked immunosorbent assay, Western blot, and immunostaining in isolated and stimulated fibroblast derived from nasal mucosa and NP from both aspirin-tolerant and aspirin-intolerant patients. The 3 methods confirmed the low expression of Cox-2 expression in NP from both aspirin-tolerant and aspirin-intolerant patients.[41]

The expression of the 4 PGE$_2$ G protein-coupled receptors designated EP$_1$ to EP$_4$ has been assessed in CRSwNP. A reduced expression of EP$_2$ receptor has been reported in nasal inflammatory cells and fibroblast of NP of aspirin-intolerant patients.[41,43,49]

Because most of the antiinflammatory effects of $PGE_2$ seem to be induced by the stimulation of the $EP_2$ receptor,[37,38] the association of the reduced release of $PGE_2$, a substance with antiinflammatory properties in the airways, with the low expression of the $PGE_2$ receptor involved in the transmission of antiinflammatory signals might contribute to the intensification of the inflammatory process in the upper airways of patients with NP, especially in those with associated aspirin intolerance.[41]

**Lipoxygenase pathway** Some studies have reported increased production of CysLT in CRSwNP of patients with asthma with and without aspirin hypersensitivity.[50] When the production of CysLT is assessed by measuring the urinary levels of leukotriene $E_4$, various studies have reported a significant higher urinary excretion of $LTE_4$ at baseline in patients with CRSwNP and aspirin intolerance compared with CRSwNP from aspirin-tolerant patients.[50] The baseline levels increase even further when aspirin-intolerant patients are challenged with oral, intravenous, and intranasal aspirin.[50–52] One recent study reported that severe aspirin-tolerant asthmatics also showed a significantly higher urinary $LTE_4$ concentration at baseline, compared with mild/moderate patients with aspirin-tolerant asthma.[53] This observation suggests that overproduction of CysLTs is closely associated with asthma severity and the presence of CRSwNP. Therefore, an increased production of CysLTs should not be considered a condition exclusively associated with aspirin hypersensitivity. Because most patients with aspirin-intolerant asthma suffer from a severe form of the disease,[10] it is possible that the increased production of CysLT production detected in these patients is related, at least in part, to the severity of the associated asthma.

A recent study found a significant decrease in the urinary $LTE_4$ concentrations after endoscopic sinus surgery in both CRSwNP aspirin-tolerant and CRSwNP aspirin-intolerant patients with asthma, probably as a consequence of the elimination of many CysLT-producing cells in the sinus.[53] This observation suggests that CRSwNP is one of the most important factors involved in CysLT overproduction in asthma.[50]

The increased production of CysLT in CRSwNP is associated with the increased expression of the $LTC_4$ synthase enzyme, and both CysLT production and $LTC_4$ synthase expression are significantly correlated with the intensity of the eosinophilic infiltration present in NP tissue.[25,43] CysLT levels in patients with CRSwNP positively correlate with IL-5 concentrations, a cytokine that primes eosinophils and thereby increases the biosynthesis capacity of these cells to produce CysLT.[25] These observations suggest that there is a close link between CysLT overproduction and the accumulation of activated eosinophil in CRSwNP.[50]

Pharmacologic studies in human individuals provide evidence for the existence of at least 3 functional receptors for CysLT, although only 2 have been identified: the so-called $CysLT_1$ and $CysLT_2$ receptors.[54] $CysLT_1$ has been detected in eosinophils, mast cells, macrophages, neutrophils and vascular cell in human nasal mucosa. $CysLT_2$ receptors are broadly distributed in leukocytes, heart tissue, brain, adrenal gland, and the vasculature.[54]

Increased numbers of nasal inflammatory cells expressing $CysLT_1$ have been reported in CRSwNP of patients with aspirin intolerance.[43,49] Desensitization with lysine-aspirin selectively reduced the number of leukocytes expressing $CysLT_1$, suggesting that downregulation of $CysLT_1$ could be a mechanism of therapeutic benefit.[55]

A recent study has also reported an increased expression of $CysLT_2$ receptor in NP from aspirin-intolerant patients with asthma compared with aspirin-tolerant asthmatics.[43] Because no data on the role of $CysLT_2$ receptor in asthma and rhinitis have been reported, the biological significance of this observation is not clear.

**Transcellular metabolisms (LXs)** Levels of $LXA_4$ have been reported as being higher in patients with CRSwNP compared with control nasal mucosa, but lower in CRSwNP of aspirin-intolerant patients compared with the levels found in CRSwNP of aspirin-tolerant asthmatics.[25] A recent study reported that the urinary levels of 15-epi-$LXA_4$ were significantly lower in aspirin-intolerant asthmatics compared with aspirin-tolerant patients and control nasal mucosa. These findings seem to indicate a deficient regulation of antiinflammatory AA metabolites generated through the transcellular pathway in patients with CRSwNP and aspirin intolerance.

Several observations support the notion that changes in the regulation of AA metabolism are involved in the path physiology of CRSwNP, especially when CRSwNP is associated with aspirin intolerance. Some studies have reported changes at different levels of the Cox pathway, including very low production of $PGE_2$, alterations in the regulation of both Cox-1 and Cox-2 under inflammatory conditions, and low expression of the $EP_2$ receptor. Moreover, studies have shown that the 5-LO pathway is very active in CRSwNP, especially when CRSwNP is associated with aspirin intolerance, resulting in an increased production of CysLTs. In contrast with $EP_2$ receptor, the CysLTs receptor $CysLT_1$ is unregulated in CRSwNP, and this helps maximize the proinflammatory effects of CysLT.

The impaired regulation of substances ($PGE_2$) and receptors ($EP_2$) with antiinflammatory effects, associated with the increased production of proinflammatory products (CysLT) and upregulation of their receptors ($CysLT_1$) probably plays a part in enhancing and perpetuating the inflammatory process present in CRSwNP. Alterations in the AA metabolisms might also contribute to the development of AERD. The mechanisms involved in the reported altered regulation of AA metabolism remain to be clarified.

# DIAGNOSIS
## CRS

The diagnosis of CRS with or without NP is based on clinical history (presence and duration for more than 12 weeks of sinonasal symptoms), nasal endoscopy (when available), and CT scan of the paranasal sinuses.[1–3] Computed axial tomography is the accepted gold standard for identifying pacifications within the sinuses, with a pattern ranging from bilateral mucosal thickening to complete opacification of all sinuses.

## AERD

The diagnosis of aspirin hypersensitivity is based on a history of adverse respiratory reactions precipitated by the intake of aspirin or other NSAIDs. In asthmatic patients with CRS and NP and a negative history or in those who have never been exposed to NSAIDs, provocation testing may be required.[56]

The reference standard for the diagnosis of hypersensitivity to aspirin and other NSAIDs is outlined in detail in the article on "AERD: clinical disease and diagnosis" elsewhere in this issue. The oral aspirin challenge and several protocols have been developed and described.[57] In Europe, inhalation (bronchial) challenge with lysine-aspirin (a soluble form of acetylsalicylic acid) was introduced more than 30 years ago[58] and is considered the test of choice for confirming or excluding aspirin sensitivity in patients with bronchial asthma. Although both tests have similar sensitivity and specificity, the inhalation test is faster and safer to perform than the oral challenge, and the adverse reaction it creates can be easily reversed with nebulized $\beta_2$ agonists. A nasal provocation test with lysine-aspirin is also a reliable tool for diagnosing aspirin hypersensitivity, providing that the clinical symptoms are combined with an objective and standardized technique of nasal airflow measurement.[59,60] The nasal test is rapid and safe and can be performed in an outpatient setting even in asthmatic patients with reduced pulmonary function who are suitable for bronchial provocation. In experienced hands, the sensitivity of intranasal aspirin provocation easily approaches the performance of the bronchial challenge.

In vitro tests measuring aspirin-specific peripheral blood leukocyte activation have recently been proposed for the diagnosis of aspirin sensitivity. These newly developed in vitro tests, involving either peripheral blood leukocytes (Aspirin-Sensitive Patients Identification Test)[61] or basophil activation[62] seem to show promising performance, but require further investigation and validation before becoming routine tools for confirming the presence of aspirin hypersensitivity.

## MANAGEMENT

The management of patients with CRSwNP and AERD is mainly based on patient training, NSAID avoidance, standard medical or surgical treatment of CRS and nasal polyposis, in addition to standard medical treatment of bronchial asthma, and potential aspirin desensitization in selected patients. The treatment also depends on the stage and severity of the disease.[1,63]

### Education and Drug Avoidance

Because aspirin and other NSAIDs can induce severe asthma attacks, the avoidance of these drugs by aspirin-sensitive patients, and their training in this respect, is a hallmark of the management of patients with CRS, NP, and AERD. Physicians should educate patients on various fronts so that they can better understand their disease: first, respiratory problems are not limited to a specific drug but they may appear after the intake of aspirin or any NSAID; second, many compounds for the common cold or flu contain aspirin or other NSAIDs and should be avoided; and third, when analgesic and antipyretic treatment is needed, several safe drugs may be recommended as alternatives, including acetaminophen (up to 1000 mg) and partially selective (meloxicam, nimesulide) or selective COX-2 inhibitors (coxibs).[64]

### Medical Treatment

Intranasal corticosteroids[1,65] and, occasionally, short courses of oral steroids[66,67] are the most effective drugs for treating CRSwNP and constitute the first line of treatment.[1,63] Both topical and systemic corticosteroids may affect the eosinophil function by both directly reducing eosinophil viability and activation or indirectly reducing the secretion of chemotactic cytokines by nasal mucosa and polyp epithelial cells, in both aspirin-sensitive and aspirin-tolerant patients.[63] For safety purposes, and because a patient with AERD receives long-term treatment with intranasal and inhaled steroids as well as short courses of oral steroids during their life span, those intranasal corticosteroids with lower drug bioavailability should be preferred.[68] Furthermore, topical corticosteroids in nasal drop formulation have shown greater efficacy than those in spray formulation in reducing the need for surgery in patients with severe CRSwNP.[69]

Other medications have proved effective for patients with CRSwNP. Nasal saline irrigation, both isotonic and hypertonic, as well as short-term (before surgery) and long-term (after surgery) antibiotics may help to alleviate nasal symptoms.[1,70] Although antileukotrienes do have some effect, they have not proved more effective in aspirin-sensitive than in aspirin-tolerant patients.[71]

Several drugs have been investigated in terms of their efficacy in the treatment of CRSwNP (**Table 1**).[1] Although some products have not shown any real efficacy (antihistamines, antimycotics, phytotherapy, capsaicin, nasal decongestants, mucolytics, topical antibiotics, and proton pump inhibitors), others have shown some efficacy but need more investigation to warrant a full recommendation in international guidelines: antileukotrienes, anti-IgE/omalizumab,[72,73] or anti-IL-5/mepolizumab.[74]

### Surgical Treatment

Sinonasal surgery (polypectomy, functional endoscopic sinus surgery, or ethmoidectomy) is reserved for patients with severe or uncontrolled symptoms and for those with inadequate improvement despite intranasal and oral steroid therapy.[1] The aim of endoscopic sinus surgery is to improve nasal symptoms and patients' quality of life but also to reduce bronchial symptoms and requirement for asthma medications.[5] However, patients with AERD seem to respond less to surgical interventions.[75,76] Patients with CRS and NP have a high tendency to recurrence after surgery: this recurrence rate is up to 10 times higher in patients with AERD, even after endoscopic sinus surgery,[77] and patients are more likely to undergo repeated sinus surgical interventions.[16] To prevent or reduce the relapse of NP, international guidelines recommend the continuation of medical management after surgery (**Table 2**).[1,65] Intranasal corticosteroids have proved their efficacy and safety for up to 5 years of treatment after surgery.[78]

### Aspirin Desensitization

Aspirin desensitization is recommended for patients with AERD with severe corticoid-dependent asthma, those with recurrent nasal polyposis requiring more than 1

**Table 1**
**Levels of evidence and recommendations for the management of adults with CRSwNP**

| Treatment | Level/Grade of Recommendation | Relevance |
|---|---|---|
| Oral antibiotics | | |
| Short-term (<4 wk) | Ib and Ib(–), C[a] | Yes<br>Small effect |
| Long-term (≥12 wk) | III, C | Yes<br>Small effect<br>If IgE level is not increased |
| Topical corticosteroids | Ia, A | Yes |
| Oral corticosteroids | Ia, A | Yes |
| Nasal saline irrigation[b] | Ib, D | Yes<br>For symptomatic relief |
| Antileukotrienes | Ib(–), A(–) | No |
| Aspirin desensitization | II, C | Unclear |

No data of efficacy or no studies for: topical antibiotics, anti-IL-5 (unclear), anti-IgE, nasal/oral decongestants, mucolytics, phytotherapy, topical/systemic antimycotics, furosemide, immunosuppressants, capsaicin, proton pump inhibitors.
[a] One positive and 1 negative study. Therefore recommendation C.
[b] No data in single use.
*Data from* Scadding G, Hellings P, Alobid I, et al. Diagnostic tools in Rhinology EAACI position paper. Clin Transl Allergy 2011;1:2.

**Table 2**
**Levels of evidence and recommendations for the postoperative management of adults with CRSwNP**

| Treatment | Level/Grade of Recommendation | Relevance |
|---|---|---|
| Oral antibiotics | | |
|   Short-term (<4 wk) | Ib, A | Yes<br>Small effect |
|   Long-term (≥12 wk) | Ib, C[a] | Yes<br>If IgE level is not increased |
| Topical corticosteroids | Ia, A | Yes |
| Oral corticosteroids | Ia, A | Yes |
| Anti-IL-5 | Ib, A | Yes |
| Anti-leukotrienes | Ib(−), A(−)[b] | No |

No data of efficacy or no studies for: oral antihistamines in allergic patients (unclear), nasal saline irrigation (unclear), anti-IgE (unclear), aspirin desensitization, furosemide.

[a] Indications exist for better efficacy in CRS without NP.

[b] Negative study, recommended not to use.

*Data from* Scadding G, Hellings P, Alobid I, et al. Diagnostic tools in Rhinology EAACI position paper. Clin Transl Allergy 2011;1:2.

operative intervention, and for patients who require aspirin or NSAID daily therapy for other medical reasons, such as chronic arthritis or coronary artery disease. Although the mechanism of action is still unclear, systemic[57,79,80] or intranasal[81,82] aspirin desensitization plays a part in protecting against recurrences of CRSwNP. Aspirin desensitization not only improves nasal symptoms such as the loss of smell but also leads to significant reductions in sinus infections, polyp formation, recurrence rate, need for polyp operations per year, and dosage of intranasal corticosteroids. See the article elsewhere in this issue for a detailed discussion of this subject.

## REFERENCES

1. Fokkens WJ, Lund V, Mullol J, et al. EPOS 2012: European position paper on rhinosinusitis and nasal polyps 2012. Rhinology 2012;50(Suppl 23):1–298.
2. Fokkens WJ, Lund V, Mullol J, et al. EPOS 2012: European position paper on rhinosinusitis and nasal polyps 2012. A summary for otorhinolaryngologists. Rhinology 2012;50(1):1–12.
3. Scadding G, Hellings P, Alobid I, et al. Diagnostic tools in Rhinology EAACI position paper. Clin Transl Allergy 2011;1:2.
4. Mullol J, Mariño-Sánchez F, Alobid I, et al. Clinical examination and differential diagnosis in rhinology. In: Georgalas C, Fokkens WJ, editors. Rhinology and skull base surgery: from the lab to the operating room. Stuttgart (Germany): Thieme; 2012. p. 134–55.
5. Awad OG, Lee JH, Fasano MB, et al. Sinonasal outcomes after endoscopic sinus surgery in asthmatic patients with nasal polyps: a difference between aspirin-tolerant and aspirin-induced asthma? Laryngoscope 2008;118(7):1282–6.
6. Robinson JL, Griest S, James KE, et al. Impact of aspirin intolerance on outcomes of sinus surgery. Laryngoscope 2007;117(5):825–30.
7. Hastan D, Fokkens WJ, Bachert C, et al. Chronic rhinosinusitis in Europe–an underestimated disease. A GA²LEN study. Allergy 2011;66(9):1216–23.

8. Kaliner MA, Osguthorpe JD, Fireman P, et al. Sinusitis: bench to bedside. Current findings, future directions. J Allergy Clin Immunol 1997;99(6):S829–48.
9. Alobid I, Cardelús S, Benítez P, et al. The impact of asthma on the sense of smell in patients with chronic rhinosinusitis and nasal polyps. Rhinology 2011;49(5):519–24.
10. Szczeklik A, Nizankowska E, Duplaga M. On behalf of the AIANE (European Network on Aspirin-Induced Asthma) Investigators. Natural history of aspirin-induced asthma. Eur Respir J 2000;16:432–6.
11. Guilemany JM, Angrill J, Alobid I, et al. United airways: the impact of chronic rhinosinusitis and nasal polyps in bronchiectasic patient's quality of life. Allergy 2009;64:1524–9.
12. Widal MF, Abrami P, Lermoyez J. Anaphylaxie et idiosyncrasie. Presse Med 1922; 30:189–92 [in French].
13. Samter M, Beers RF Jr. Intolerance to aspirin. Clinical studies and consideration of its pathogenesis. Ann Intern Med 1968;68(5):975–83.
14. Bavbek S, Dursun B, Dursun E, et al. The prevalence of aspirin hypersensitivity in patients with nasal polyposis and contributing factors. Am J Rhinol Allergy 2011; 25(6):411–5.
15. Settipane GA, Chafee FH. Nasal polyps in asthma and rhinitis. A review of 6,037 patients. J Allergy Clin Immunol 1977;59(1):17–21.
16. Vento SI, Ertama LO, Hytönen ML, et al. Nasal polyposis: clinical course during 20 years. Ann Allergy Asthma Immunol 2000;85(3):209–14.
17. Alobid I, Bernal-Sprekelsen M, Mullol J. Chronic rhinosinusitis and nasal polyps. The role of generic and specific questionnaires on assessing its impact on patient's quality of life. Allergy 2008;63(10):1267–79.
18. Alobid I, Benítez P, Valero A, et al. The impact of atopy, sinus opacification, and nasal patency on quality of life in patients with severe nasal polyposis. Otolaryngol Head Neck Surg 2006;134:609–12.
19. Alobid I, Benítez P, Bernal-Sprekelsen M, et al. The impact of asthma and aspirin sensitivity on quality of life of patients with nasal polyposis. Qual Life Res 2005;14: 789–93.
20. Alobid I, Benítez P, Bernal-Sprekelsen M, et al. Nasal polyposis and its impact on quality of life. Comparison between the effects of medical and surgical treatments. Allergy 2005;60:452–8.
21. Pleis JR, Lucas JW, Ward BW. Summary health statistics for U.S. adults: National Health Interview Survey, 2008. Vital Health Stat 10 2009;(242):1–157.
22. Bhattacharyya N, Orlandi RR, Grebner J, et al. Cost burden of chronic rhinosinusitis: a claims-based study. Otolaryngol Head Neck Surg 2011;144(3):440–5.
23. Berges-Gimeno MP, Simon RA, Stevenson DD. The natural history and clinical characteristics of aspirin-exacerbated respiratory disease. Ann Allergy Asthma Immunol 2002;89(5):474–8.
24. Bachert C, Gevaert P, Holtappels G, et al. Nasal polyposis: from cytokines to growth. Am J Rhinol 2000;14:279–90.
25. Pérez-Novo C, Watelet JB, Claeys C, et al. Prostaglandin, leukotriene, and lipoxin balance in chronic rhinosinusitis with and without nasal polyposis. J Allergy Clin Immunol 2005;115:1189–96.
26. Zang N, van Zele T, Pérez-Novo C, et al. Different types of T-effector cells orchestrated mucosal inflammation in chronic sinus disease. J Allergy Clin Immunol 2008;122:961–8.
27. Beck LA, Stellato C, Beall LD, et al. Detection of the chemokine RANTES and endothelial adhesion molecules in nasal polyps. J Allergy Clin Immunol 1996; 98:766–80.

28. Olze H, Forster U, Zuberbier T, et al. Eosinophilic nasal polyps are rich source of eotaxin-1, eotaxin-2 and eotaxin-3. Rhinology 2006;44:145–50.
29. Pods R, Ross D, van Hulst S, et al. RANTES, eotaxin and eotaxin-2 expression and production in patients with aspirin triad. Allergy 2003;58:1165–70.
30. Jahsen FL, Haraldsen G, Aanesen JP, et al. Eosinophilic infiltration is related to increased expression of vascular adhesion molecule-1 in nasal polyps. Am J Respir Cell Mol Biol 1995;12:624–32.
31. Van Zele T, Claeys S, Gevaert P, et al. Differentiation of chronic sinus diseases by measurement of inflammatory mediators. Allergy 2006;61:1280–9.
32. Kowalski ML, Lewnansowska-Polak A, Wozniak J, et al. Association of stem cell factor expression in nasal polyp epithelial cells with aspirin sensitivity and asthma. Allergy 2005;60:613–7.
33. Simmons DL, Botting RM, Hla T. Cyclooxygnease isoenzymes: the biology of prostaglandin synthesis and inhibition. Pharmacol Rev 2004;56:387–437.
34. Siegle I, Klein T, Backman JT, et al. Expression of cyclooxygenase 2 in human synovial tissue. Differential elevation of cyclooxygenase 2 in inflammatory joint diseases. Arthritis Rheum 1998;41:122–9.
35. Roca-Ferrer J, Pujols L, Gartner S, et al. Upregulation of COX-1 and COX-2 in nasal polyps in cystic fibrosis. Thorax 2006;61:592.
36. Xaubet A, Roca-Ferrer J, Pujols L, et al. Cyclooxygenase-2 is up-regulated in lung parenchyma of chronic obstructive pulmonary disease and down-regulated in idiopathic pulmonary fibrosis. Sarcoidosis Vasc Diffuse Lung Dis 2004;21:35–42.
37. Vancheri C, Mastruzzo C, Sortino MA, et al. The lung as a privileged site for the beneficial actions of $PGE_2$. Trends Immunol 2004;25:40–6.
38. Sugimoto Y, Narumiya S. Prostaglandin E receptors. J Biol Chem 2007;282: 11613–7.
39. Picado C. Mechanisms of aspirin sensitivity. Curr Allergy Asthma Rep 2006;6: 198–202.
40. Kanaoka Y, Boyce JA. Cysteinyl leukotrienes and their receptors: cellular distribution and function in immune and inflammatory responses. J Immunol 2004;173: 1503–10.
41. Roca-Ferrer J, Garcia-Garcia FJ, Pereda J, et al. Reduced expression of COXs and production of prostaglandin E2 in patients with nasal polyps with and without aspirin-intolerant asthma. J Allergy Clin Immunol 2011;128:66–72.
42. Picado C, Fernández-Morata JC, Juan M, et al. Cyclooxygenase-2 mRNA is downexpressed in nasal polyps from aspirin-sensitive asthmatics. Am J Respir Crit Care Med 1999;160:291–6.
43. Adamusiak AM, Stasikowska-Kanicka O, Lewandowska-Polak A, et al. Expression of arachidonate metabolisms enzymes and receptors in nasal polyps of aspirin-hypersensitive asthmatics. Int Arch Allergy Immunol 2010;157:354–62.
44. Mullol J, Fernàndez-Morata JC, Roca-Ferrer J, et al. Cyclooxygenase 1 and cyclooxygenase 2 expression is abnormally regulated in human nasal polyps. J Allergy Clin Immunol 2002;109:824–30.
45. Pujols L, Mullol J, Alobid I, et al. Dynamics of COX-2 in nasal mucosa and nasal polyps from aspirin-tolerant and aspirin-intolerant patients with asthma. J Allergy Clin Immunol 2004;114:814–9.
46. Picado C, Bioque G, Roca-Ferrer J, et al. Nuclear factor-kappa C activity is downregulated in nasal polyps from aspirin-sensitive asthmatics. Allergy 2003;58:122–6.
47. Adamjee J, Suh YJ, Park HS, et al. Expression of 5-lipoxygenase and cyclooxygenase pathway enzymes in nasal polyps of patients with aspirin-intolerant asthma. J Pathol 2006;209:392–9.

48. Sampson AP. Aspirin-intolerant asthma. New insights from bronchial mucosal biopsies. In: Sczceklik A, Gryglewski RJ, Vane J, editors. Eicosanoids, aspirin and asthma. New York: Marcel Dekker; 1998. p. 371–89.
49. Ying S, Meng Q, Scadding G, et al. Aspirin-sensitive rhinosinusitis is associated with reduced E-prostanoid 2 receptor expression on nasal mucosal inflammatory cells. J Allergy Clin Immunol 2006;117:312–8.
50. Higashi N, Taniguchi M, Mita H, et al. Aspirin-intolerant asthma (AIA) assessment using the urinary biomarkers, leukotrine $E_4$ (LTE$_4$) and prostaglandin $E_2$ (PGD$_2$) metabolites. Allergol Int 2012;61:393–403.
51. Micheletto C, Tognella S, Visconti M, et al. Changes in urinary LTE4 and nasal functions following nasal provocation test with ASA in ASA-tolerant and-intolerant asthmatics. Respir Med 2006;100:2144–50.
52. Picado C, Ramis I, Rosello J, et al. Release of peptide leukotriene into nasal secretions after local instillation of aspirin in aspirin-sensitive asthmatic patients. Am Rev Respir Dis 1992;145:1028–9.
53. Higashi N, Taniguchi M, Mita H, et al. Clinical features of asthmatic patients with increased urinary leukotriene $E_4$ excretion (hyperleukotrienuria): involvement of chronic hyperplastic rhinosinusitis with nasal polyposis. J Allergy Clin Immunol 2004;113:277–83.
54. Laidlaw TM, Boyc JA. Cysteinyl leukotriene receptors, old and new: implications for asthma. Clin Exp Allergy 2012;42:1313–20.
55. Sousa AR, Parikh A, Scadding G, et al. Leukotriene-receptor expression on nasal mucosal inflammatory cells in aspirin-sensitive rhinosinusitis. N Engl J Med 2002; 347:1493–9.
56. Nizankowska-Mogilnicka E, Bochenek G, Mastalerz L, et al. EAACI/GA2LEN guideline: aspirin provocation tests for diagnosis of aspirin hypersensitivity. Allergy 2007;62(10):1111–8.
57. Stevenson DD. Aspirin sensitivity and desensitization for asthma and sinusitis. Curr Allergy Asthma Rep 2009;9(2):155–63.
58. Bianco SR, Robuschi M, Petrini G. Aspirin induced tolerance in aspirin asthma detected by a new challenge test. IRCS J Med Sci 1977;5:129.
59. Milewski M, Mastalerz L, Nizankowska E, et al. Nasal provocation test with lysine-aspirin for diagnosis of aspirin-sensitive asthma. J Allergy Clin Immunol 1998; 101(5):581–6.
60. Casadevall J, Ventura PJ, Mullol J, et al. Intranasal challenge with aspirin in the diagnosis of aspirine-intolerant asthma. Evaluation of nasal response by acoustic rhinometry. Thorax 2000;55:921–4.
61. Kowalski ML, Ptasinska A, Jedrzejczak M, et al. Aspirin-triggered 15-HETE generation in peripheral blood leukocytes is a specific and sensitive Aspirin-Sensitive Patients Identification Test (ASPITest). Allergy 2005;60(9):1139–45.
62. Kim MS, Cho YJ. Flow cytometry-assisted basophil activation test as a safe diagnostic tool for aspirin/NSAID hypersensitivity. Allergy Asthma Immunol Res 2012; 4(3):137–42.
63. Alobid I, Mullol J. Role of medical therapy in the management of nasal polyps. Curr Allergy Asthma Rep 2012;12(1):144–53.
64. Kowalski ML, Makowska J. Use of nonsteroidal anti-inflammatory drugs in patients with aspirin hypersensitivity: safety of cyclo-oxygenase-2 inhibitors. Treat Respir Med 2006;5(6):399–406.
65. Mullol J, Obando A, Pujols L, et al. Corticosteroid treatment in chronic rhinosinusitis: the possibilities and the limits. Immunol Allergy Clin North Am 2009;29(4): 657–68.

66. Mullol J, Alobid I. Combined oral and intranasal corticosteroid therapy: an advance in the management of nasal polyposis? Ann Intern Med 2011;154(5): 365–7.
67. Martinez-Devesa P, Patiar S. Oral steroids for nasal polyps. Cochrane Database Syst Rev 2011;(7):CD005232.
68. Derendorf H, Meltzer EO. Molecular and clinical pharmacology of intranasal corticosteroids: clinical and therapeutic implications. Allergy 2008;63(10):1292–300.
69. Aukema AA, Mulder PG, Fokkens WJ. Treatment of nasal polyposis and chronic rhinosinusitis with fluticasone propionate nasal drops reduces need for sinus surgery. J Allergy Clin Immunol 2005;115:1017–23.
70. Van Zele T, Gevaert P, Holtappels G, et al. Oral steroids and doxycycline: two different approaches to treat nasal polyps. J Allergy Clin Immunol 2010;125(5): 1069–1076.e4.
71. Ragab S, Parikh A, Darby YC, et al. An open audit of montelukast, a leukotriene receptor antagonist, in nasal polyposis associated with asthma. Clin Exp Allergy 2001;31:1385–91.
72. Vennera MC, Picado C, Mullol J, et al. Efficacy of omalizumab in the treatment of nasal polyps. Thorax 2011;66(9):824–5.
73. Gevaert P, Calus L, Van Zele T, et al. Omalizumab is effective in allergic and nonallergic patients with nasal polyps and asthma. J Allergy Clin Immunol 2012. http://dx.doi.org/10.1016/j.jaci.2012.07.047.
74. Gevaert P, Van Bruaene N, Cattaert T, et al. Mepolizumab, a humanized anti-IL-5 mAb, as a treatment option for severe nasal polyposis. J Allergy Clin Immunol 2011;128(5):989–995.e1-8.
75. Batra PS, Kern RC, Tripathi A, et al. Outcome analysis of endoscopic sinus surgery in patients with nasal polyps and asthma. Laryngoscope 2003;113(10): 1703–6.
76. Mendelsohn D, Jeremic G, Wright ED, et al. Revision rates after endoscopic sinus surgery: a recurrence analysis. Ann Otol Rhinol Laryngol 2011;120(3):162–6.
77. Kim JE, Kountakis SE. The prevalence of Samter's triad in patients undergoing functional endoscopic sinus surgery. Ear Nose Throat J 2007;86(7):396–9.
78. Rowe-Jones JM, Medcalf M, Durham SR, et al. Functional endoscopic sinus surgery: 5 year follow up and results of a prospective, randomised, stratified, double-blind, placebo controlled study of postoperative fluticasone propionate aqueous nasal spray. Rhinology 2005;43(1):2–10.
79. Nucera E, Schiavino D, Milani A, et al. Effects of lysine-acetylsalicylate (LAS) treatment in nasal polyposis: two controlled long term prospective follow up studies. Thorax 2000;55:75–8.
80. Pfaar O, Klimek L. Eicosanoids, aspirin-intolerance and the upper airways–current standards and recent improvements of the desensitization therapy. J Physiol Pharmacol 2006;57(Suppl 12):5–13.
81. Parikh AA, Scadding GK. Intranasal lysine-aspirin in aspirin-sensitive nasal polyposis: a controlled trial. Laryngoscope 2005;115:1385–90.
82. Ogata N, Darby Y, Scadding G. Intranasal lysine-aspirin administration decreases polyp volume in patients with aspirin-intolerant asthma. J Laryngol Otol 2007;121:1156–60.

# Genetics of Hypersensitivity to Aspirin and Nonsteroidal Anti-inflammatory Drugs

Seung-Hyun Kim, PhD[a], Marek Sanak, MD, PhD[a,b], Hae-Sim Park, MD, PhD[a,*]

## KEYWORDS

- Genetic association • Hypersensitivity • Nonsteroidal anti-inflammatory drugs

## KEY POINTS

- Persistent inflammation with marked inflammatory cell activation, unbalanced leukotriene production, and enhanced biochemical signaling cascades may be important pathogenic mechanisms underlying aspirin hypersensitivity.
- Epigenetic factors, heterogeneous inflammatory cells, and interindividual variability in drug metabolism combined with variations in immunologic backgrounds should also be considered as underlying mechanisms.
- Biologic and/or functional studies should be performed for a further comprehensive understanding of the complex etiology of aspirin hypersensitivity.

Given the universality of aspirin and other nonsteroidal anti-inflammatory drug (NSAID) administration for their analgesic and antipyretic activities, various hypersensitivity reactions have been reported. Hypersensitivty can occur regardless of a chemical drug structure or its therapeutic potency. The most common allergic conditions are aspirin-exacerbated respiratory disease (AERD or aspirin-induced asthma),[1,2] aspirin-induced urticaria/angioedema (AIU),[3] the both together named blended reaction, and in rare cases, anaphylaxis.[4]

Several genetic studies on aspirin hypersensitivity have been performed to discover the genetic predisposition to aspirin hypersensitivity and to gain insight into the phenotypic diversity. This article updates data on the genetic mechanisms that govern AERD and AIU and summarizes recent findings on the molecular genetic mechanism of aspirin hypersensitivity.

This work was supported by a grant of the Korean Health 21 R&D project, Ministry of Health and Welfare, ROK (A111218-11-PG01).

The authors have nothing to disclose.

[a] Department of Allergy & Clinical Immunology, Ajou University School of Medicine, San-5, Woncheondong, Youngtonggu, Suwon 442-721, Republic of Korea; [b] Division of Molecular Biology and Clinical Genetics, Department of Medicine, Jagiellonian University Medical College, 8 Skawinska Street, Krakow 31-066, Poland

* Corresponding author.

E-mail address: hspark@ajou.ac.kr

Immunol Allergy Clin N Am 33 (2013) 177–194
http://dx.doi.org/10.1016/j.iac.2012.10.003
0889-8561/13/$ – see front matter © 2013 Elsevier Inc. All rights reserved.

## HISTORICAL REVIEW OF GENETIC STUDIES ON ASPIRIN HYPERSENSITIVITY

Many genetic association studies have been performed in recent years to understand the genetic basis of aspirin hypersensitivity. Candidate gene association studies have been performed as case–control studies by comparing the frequencies of candidate gene polymorphisms between case and control groups.

### Candidate Gene Approaches to Aspirin Hypersensitivity

#### Arachidonic acid metabolism

The rationale for targeting arachidonic acid metabolism-related genes based on the cyclooxygenase (COX) theory.[5] Previous studies demonstrated that the inhibitory action of aspirin and other NSAIDs on COX enzyme activity resulted in cysteinyl leukotriene (CysLT) overproduction, which is a biomarker of AERD.[6,7] The first genetic studies were reported in 1997 and focused on 5-lipoxygenase (5-LO; ALOX5)[8] and leukotriene C4 synthase (LTC4S)[9] genes. These studies indicated that functional variants in the ALOX5 and LTC4S genes modify transcriptional regulation through altered transcription factor-binding affinities. LTC4 synthase is a critical enzyme in leukotriene production.[10] Increased expression of LTC4S associated with LTC4S gene (-444A>C) promoter polymorphism could affect susceptibility to aspirin hypersensitivity.[11] The genetic contribution of the LTC4S-444 promoter polymorphism is supported by increased LTC4S mRNA expression in blood eosinophils,[11] bronchial mucosa,[12] bronchial mast cells,[13] and nasal mucosa[14] in patients with AERD. ALOX5 gene expression is genetically regulated, particularly by a variable number of tandem repeats (VNTRs) of Sp1 binding motif in the promoter region.[8] VNTR of ALOX5 is also associated with the severity of airway hyper-responsiveness in patients with AERD[15] and response to leukotriene receptor antagonists (LTRA)[16] The proinflammatory effect of CysLTs may be affected by genetic variants of their receptors. A cysteinyl leukotriene receptor 1 (CysLTR1) gene polymorphism has been identified in a Korean population,[17] in which 3 promoter polymorphisms (−634C>T, −475A>C, and −336A>G) modulate CysLTR1 gene expression to increase AERD susceptibility. This is consistent with a previous finding of increased CysLTR1 expression in nasal mucosa inflammatory cells from patients with AERD.[18] Moreover, the CysLTR1 promoter polymorphism also shows a pharmacogenetic effect on LTRA therapy.[19] A second receptor, CysLTR2, has been identified as a genetic risk factor[20] in which genetic variants have affected the transcription and stability of the CysLTR2 mRNA. CysLTs mediate bronchocontriction, mucus hypersecretion, and microvascular leakage via CysLTR1. This receptor has the highest high-affinity for LTD4, whereas CysLTR2 also mediates the inflammatory response, vascular permeability, and tissue fibrosis, showing an equal affinity for LTC4 and LTD4.[10,21] The third CysLT receptor, which may include G protein-coupled receptor 17 (GPR17) and purinergic receptor (P2Y)-like receptor, has been proposed to contribute in airway inflammation and eosinophil activation[22]; however, no genetic studies were reported.

A functional promoter polymorphism of the COX-2 gene (−765G>C) has been identified in a Polish population[23] in which the variant could contribute to increase prostaglandin (PG) D2 production in patients with AERD. Downstream the pathway of prostaglandins, Jinnai and colleagues[24] reported a functional single nucleotide polymorphism (SNP) (μS5) located in the regulatory region of the PGE2 receptor subtype 2 gene (PTGER2, EP2) as a genetic risk factor, and the variant may contribute to the reduced protective effect of PGE2 by a decreased transcription activity. These findings are consistent with previous reports of decreased COX-2 expression in nasal polyps[25] and decreased PGE2 production in nasal epithelial cells from patients with

AERD.[7] Four PGE2 receptors with different tissue distributions may play important roles in the pathogenesis of AERD by mediating the PGE2 signal.[26,27] Several studies have demonstrated that other genetic variations in the prostanoid receptors (PTGER2, PTGER3, PTGER4, PTGIR) are strongly associated with the AERD phenotype.[24,28,29] Also in the COX pathway, thromboxane A2 has been considered an important mediator, because it can induce bronchoconstriction and hyper-responsiveness, which are typical features of asthma.[30] Thromboxane A synthase 1 (TBXAS1) catalyzes the conversion of PGH2 to thromboxane A2, and the genotypic variant of the *TBXAS1* gene (rs6962291) may play a protective role in the development of AERD by reducing catalytic activity of the gene.[31] A genetic polymorphism of the thromboxane receptor (TBXA2R) increases the bronchoconstrictive response to aspirin in patients with AERD.[32,33]

Among other arachidonate metabolites, 15-hydroxyeicosatetranoic (15-HETE) is a key biomarker involved in AERD pathogenesis, as evidenced by increased generation of 15-HETE in peripheral blood leukocytes from patients with AERD.[34] Therefore, it can be suggested as a potential diagnostic biomarker for in vitro diagnostics of AERD. 15-Lipoxygenase (ALOX15) plays an important role during 15-HETE synthesis by catalyzing the conversion of arachidonic acid to 15-hydroxyperoxyeicosatetranoic acid (15-HPETE) and 15-HETE, which act as anti-inflammatory mediators and functional antagonists of leukotrienes.[6] Polymorphisms of the *ALOX15* gene could affect enzyme activity by modulating transcriptional regulation, ultimately leading to genetic susceptibility to AERD. The effect of *ALOX15* variants seems related to the total eosinophil count in patients with AERD.[35] Both lipoxin LXA4 and aspirin-triggered 15-epi lipoxin 4 play regulatory roles in leukocyte trafficking and inflammatory responses through the formyl peptide receptor (FPR2, also known as FPRL1, ALXR).[36] A recent candidate genetic study demonstrated that the variant of the *FPR2* gene (-4209T>G) may have a protective role in the development of AERD by modulating FPR2 protein expression.[37] Other 15-HPETE products include eoxins (EXs). EXA4 can be conjugated with glutathione, leading to the formation of cysteinyl leukotrenes analogs: EXC4, EXD4, and EXE4. Eoxins, produced in 15-LO pathway, may contribute to inflammation in patients with AERD due to eosinophil infiltration and activation within airways.[38]

Cutaneous hypersensitivity reactions to aspirin and NSAIDs often occur in the form of urticaria and angioedema. Although the genetic mechanisms of the cutaneous response to aspirin are poorly understood, several reports have suggested that overproduction of cysteinyl leukotrienes may be involved.[3,39] Mastalerz and colleagues[40] demonstrated leukotriene overproduction in association with the *LTC4S* promoter polymorphism (–444A>C) in patients with aspirin-induced urticaria/angioedema (AIU). Moreover, AIU aggregated in 2 families inheriting the *LTC4S* –444C allele.[41] Among the 4 leukotriene-related genes, including *ALOX5*, 5-lipoxygenase-activating protein (*ALOX5AP*), COX-2 (*PTGS2*), and *CYSLTR1*, the frequency of the *CYSLTR1*– 634T allele is significantly lower in patients with aspirin-intolerant chronic urticaria (AICU) than that in those with AERD groups,[42] suggesting that the *CYSLTR1* gene polymorphism contribution can vary with the 2 major aspirin-related phenotypes in the Korean population.

*Effector function of inflammatory cells during chronic inflammation*
The key biochemical feature of AERD is increased cysteinyl leukotriene production both at baseline[43,44] and following an aspirin challenge.[45,46] Abundant sources of CysLTs include eosinophils and mast cells,[10] which are numerous in the nasal and bronchial mucosa of patients with AERD.[47,48] Several reports have addressed the

importance of inflammatory cells in patients with AERD. Increased *LTC4S* mRNA expression in various inflammatory cells such as blood eosinophils[11] and bronchial mast cells[13] has also been noted in patients with AERD. This is accompanied by increased CysLTR1 expression in nasal mucosal inflammatory cells from patients with AERD.[18] Therefore, both eosinophils and mast cells contribute to aspirin hypersensitivity by leukotriene overproduction within the airways. Both types of inflammatory cells are important effector cells during persistent inflammation in patients with AERD.

Chronic eosinophilic inflammation in the upper and lower airways is a key feature in patients with AERD[49]; therefore, eosinophilic inflammation-related genes have been screened as potential candidate genes in genetic association studies. Genetic studies on interleukin-13 (IL-13) gene polymorphisms in relation with AERD have demonstrated that the gene variants are associated with eosinophil counts and serum eotaxin-1 levels and contribute to the development of rhinosinusitis, which is an important intermediate phenotype of AERD.[50] The chemokine CC motif receptor-3 (CCR3) is an important cytokine receptor mediating eosinophil infiltration. Interestingly, *CCR3* gene mRNA expression increases significantly after aspirin provocation in patients with AERD,[51] and the promoter polymorphism is associated with the AERD phenotype. The promoter polymorphism of *CRTH2* gene encoding the chemoattractant receptor molecule expressed in Th2 cells is significantly associated with serum eotaxin-2 level in patients with AERD and contributes to eosinophilic infiltration.[33,52] IL-4 gene expression is regulated by promoter polymorphisms (–33C>T and –589C>T) through modulation of the binding affinity of transcription factors such as CCAAT/Enhancer-binding protein β (C/EBPβ) and Nuclear factor of activated T-cells (NFAT). This effect is dependent on aspirin and contributes to aspirin hypersensitivity in susceptible patients.[53]

Mast cells produce IL-4, IL-5, and IL-13 to provoke an inflammatory cascade and CysLTs and PGs to induce bronchoconstriction. Considering the importance of mast cells and their activation mechanism, immunoglobulin E (IgE) and histamine signaling-related genes have been targeted in candidate gene association studies. The promoter polymorphism of *FCER1A* encoding the alpha chain of the high-affinity IgE receptor I (–334C>T) is significantly associated with AIU and IgE-mediated histamine-release activity. The genotypic variant shows increased binding affinity of the Myc-associated zinc finger protein leading to increased gene expression.[54] Histamine is an important biogenic amine in chronic skin inflammation during AIU, and histamine level is regulated by its catabolism through histamine N-methyl transferase (HNMT). Functional variability in the *HNMT* gene based on the genetic polymorphisms in patients with AIU[55] has been reported in the Korean population, and the genetic variant of *HNMT* (939A>C) may affect mRNA stability and protein expression, resulting in decreased histamine inactivation, which contributes to the development of the AIU phenotype.

Platelets and platelet-adherent eosinophils are important effectors in the pathogenesis of AERD, in which the frequency of platelet-adherent eosinophils increases significantly both in the tissue of paranasal sinuses and in blood of patients with AERD; these intercellular aggregates have a close correlation with systemic CysLT production.[56] This finding suggests that platelets may be important for the accumulation of eosinophils and persistent inflammation in the pathogenesis of AERD. Therefore, other genes involved in platelet activation and leukocyte aggregation may be the appropriate candidates for the next studies to investigate susceptibility to AERD.

An immunohistochemical study of skin tissue from patients with AIU showed infiltration with activated neutrophils.[57] A genetic study on the IL-18 gene polymorphism suggested that the high transcriptional activity haplotype, *ht*1 [CG] of the IL-18 gene may contribute to the development of cutaneous inflammation sensitive to aspirin by increasing mRNA expression and subsequent neutrophil chemotaxis.[58]

### HLA association

Two strong HLA markers for aspirin hypersensitivity have been reported in results of case–control association studies. HLA-DPB1*0301 is associated with clinical features of AERD, such as a decline in forced expiratory volume in 1 second of expiration ($FEV_1$) after aspirin provocation and a higher prevalence of rhinosinusitis and nasal polyps.[59] This HLA allele has also been linked with a higher requirement for a leukotriene receptor antagonist to control asthma symptoms in patients with AERD,[60] whereas the HLA-DRB1*1302- DQB1*0609-DPB1*0201 haplotype is associated with the AIU phenotype.[61]

### Genome-Wide Association Studies

With the rapid progress in the genotyping technology and the expansion of the SNP database (nearly 4 million SNPs) through the international Hap-Map Consortium, high-throughput SNP genotyping across the genome has been applied to human diseases, mostly using SNP microarrays. These genotyping arrays allow to simultaneously determine more than 500,000 SNPs in the genome. This genome-wide approach is a hypothesis-free; therefore, novel genetic risk candidates involved in the pathogenesis of aspirin hypersensitivity can be discovered.

Although several genome-wide association studies (GWAS) have been performed on asthma, and several interesting genetic markers such as ORMDL3,[62] PDE4D,[63] RAD50,[64] and IL1RL1[65] have been identified and replicated in asthmatics, the only 1 GWAS has been reported on AERD in the Korean population.[66] Based on the GWAS in the first study cohort, the top 11 genetic variants were chosen for a genetic replication study in a different second cohort. A centrosomal protein CEP68 gene polymorphism was identified as a genetic risk factor. A nonsynonymous SNP of the CEP68 gene was the most strongly associated risk factor, and the variant AA genotype was also associated with a decline in $FEV_1$ after aspirin provocation. Functionally, a G to A conversion in CEP68 results in substitution of amino acids from glycine to serine, which may affect protein polarity. Although the mechanism of how the CEP68 gene affects AERD phenotype remains obscure, this information could provide new insights into aspirin hypersensitivity but requires functional studies of the gene. Moreover, previously identified genetic polymorphisms, particularly within 5-lipoxygenase and COX-related genes, were replicated and significantly associated with AERD in this GWAS study, even though the P value was marginal. While GWAS is a very powerful tool to discover novel disease loci, several limitations have to be overcome. A very large number of subjects (thousands within each contrasted group) should be enrolled to identify a candidate on a genome-wide significance level. GWAS results may include false positives due to multiple tests or hidden stratifications, so very stringent thresholds of significance and replication with independent samples should be used. More importantly, follow-up functional studies are essential to understand how genetic variance influences the pathogenesis of aspirin hypersensitivity.

## WHAT HAVE GENETIC STUDIES OF ASPIRIN HYPERSENSITIVITY TOLD SO FAR?

The past decades of genetic studies, which have focused on arachidonic acid metabolism (leukotrienes and PGs) in the pathogenesis of AERD, have suggested that its dysregulation leading to leukotriene overproduction and PGE2 deficiency seems to be related to the gene polymorphisms involved in the lipoxygenase and COX pathways. Genetic predisposition to abnormal leukotriene production is 1 factor underlying aspirin hypersensitivity. Other candidate gene association studies have been performed in recent years in addition to arachidonate metabolism-related studies. These candidate gene association studies have provided new insights into the pathogenesis of aspirin hypersensitivity. The genetic mechanisms that have been implicated in genetic studies on AERD are summarized in **Table 1**.

### Initiation of the Immune Response

The HLA immunocompatibility system comprises very important molecules for initiation of the immune response to foreign antigens, and several polymorphisms in the HLA region on chromosome 6 are linked with drug hypersensitivity.[67] In a survey of HLA markers specific to aspirin hypersensitivity, HLA- DPB1* 0301 was the strongest genetic marker for AERD,[59] and the HLA-DRB1*1302- DQB1*0609-DPB1*0201 haplotype was a potential genetic marker for AIU.[61] Moreover, the gene-encoding transporter 2 (TAP2), which is associated with antigen processing, is located within the major histocompatibility complex class 2 region and possesses genetic variants with a significant association to AERD-related symptoms. These symptoms include a decline in $FEV_1$ following aspirin uptake,[68,69] which represents a bronchoconstrictive reaction following aspirin ingestion.

Proteins of the inflammatory response complement cascade may be also associated with the development of AERD. During aspirin challenge, increased levels of the complement proteins C3a and C4a were observed in plasma from patients with AERD.[70] The genetic variant in the human complement component 6 (C6) gene is associated with AERD susceptibility as well as a decline in $FEV_1$ after aspirin provocation.[71] This finding suggests that complement activation, which shows an effector function for innate and adaptive immunity, may be involved in AERD pathogenesis.

Chronic viral infection has been proposed as an initiating or facilitating factor for the development of AERD.[72,73] Interestingly, a hypersensitive response to aspirin in some patients with AERD is diminished during acyclovir treatment of a herpes simplex virus infection.[74] A recent genetic study suggested an association between the toll-like receptor 3 (TLR3) gene polymorphism (-299698G>T) and the AERD phenotype.[75] As recognition that viral RNA by TLR3 can activate inflammatory signaling, functional dysregulation of TLR3 in carriers of the genetic variant can predispose asthmatics to increased AERD susceptibility. Therefore, an airway viral infection may result in persistent bronchial inflammation and increase susceptibility to aspirin or NSAIDs.

### Dysfunction of Epithelial Cells

Epithelial cells are important structural cells that regulate the inflammatory response and interact with the environment.[76] They produce and release proinflammatory cytokines and chemokines, which can prolong inflammation, finally leading to structural alterations in the epithelium. Genotypic variants in the EMID2 gene, which encodes emilin/multimerin domain-containing protein 2, show a significant effect on declines in $FEV_1$ following aspirin provocation, a key diagnostic parameter for AERD.[77] The EMID2 gene encodes the collagen XXVI α1 chain (COL26A1), a key element of extracellular matrix deposition. The serine proteinase inhibitor Kazal type 5 (SPINK5) gene encodes lymphoepithelial Kazal type-related inhibitor, an epithelial proteinase inhibitor that plays a role in the maintenance and function of epithelial cells. A genetic study demonstrated a significant association between the heterozygous SNPs G1258A and A1103G and AERD with decreased SPINK5 expression, suggesting that decreased SPINK5 expression may alter epithelial function and enhance chronic inflammation.[78] Abnormal cilia in bronchial epithelial cells may be related to respiratory disease.[79] The kinesin family number 3A (KIF3A) gene encodes a motor subunit of kinesin-2 important for cilia formation[80,81] and has been investigated in a Korean population.[82] That study found increased *KIF3A* mRNA expression in bronchial epithelial cells and protein expression in nasal polyp epithelial cells from patients with AERD. The genotypic variant of the gene is also significantly associated with AERD, as well as a decline in $FEV_1$ after aspirin provocation. These findings indicate that variations in a structural protein can influence the development of aspirin hypersensitivity.

### Biochemical Signaling of Inflammation

The anti-inflammatory action of aspirin rests primarily on its ability to inhibit COX activity, but non-COX target molecules of aspirin and NSAIDs may induce persistent inflammation. Thus, aspirin/NSAIDs may regulate a more complex network of biochemical and cellular events in inflammatory cells. Aspirin can inhibit NF-κB signaling[83] and IL-4-induced STAT6 activation[84] in various cells. Several genetic variants in the biochemical cascade of inflammation have been reported as genetic risk factors for the AERD phenotype.[85–88] Peroxisome proliferator-activated receptors are transcriptional factors that regulate the expression of genes involved in allergic inflammation and airway remodeling.[89] *PPARG* gene polymorphism *82466C>T* is associated with the development of aspirin hypersensitivity by regulating gene expression, leading to an altered response to leukotrienes.[85] The solute carrier family 6 (neurotransmitter transporter, betaine/γ-aminobutyric acid [GABA]) member 12 (*SLC6A12*) gene of the GABA signaling pathway in airway epithelium plays a critical role in asthma development through its ability to enhance mucus production.[90] The minor allele frequencies of 2 polymorphisms (*rs499368* and *rs557881*) and 1 haplotype (*SLC6A12_BL1_ht1*) are significantly associated with the risk of aspirin hypersensitivity in asthmatics, and the genotypic variants could affect the bronchoconstrictive response to aspirin and decline in $FEV_1$ following aspirin provocation.[86] An abnormal calcium-signaling pathway may induce leukotriene secretion and recruitment of inflammatory cells. A genotype variant of the voltage-dependent calcium channel gamma subunit 6 (*CACNG6*) gene (rs192808), is significantly associated with AERD,[88] suggesting voltage-dependent calcium channel and aspirin hypersensitivity in asthmatics. However, further biologic or functional evidence is needed to confirm this association.

Protein tyrosine kinases are very important signaling molecules during the activation of inflammatory cells,[91] and their inhibitors prevent airway hyper-responsiveness by reducing eosinophil infiltration into the airways.[92] A recent study reported a serine/threonine kinase 10-gene (*STK10*) polymorphism (*rs2306961 A>G, K210K*) as a genetic risk factor for AERD.[93] However, direct evidence for functional variability based on the polymorphism has not been demonstrated. The ubiquitin–proteasome pathway-related gene (*UBE3C*) polymorphisms could affect the AERD phenotype by modulating inhibitor kB (IkB) ubiquitination and suppressing nuclear factor kB (NF-kB) activation, leading to a decrease in lung function due to airway inflammation.[94] Moreover, the promoter polymorphism (rs10949635G>T) is also associated with nasal polyposis in asthmatics, which is the key feature of AERD.[95] These findings suggest that the ubiquitin–proteasome pathway may contribute to the hypersensitive response to aspirin and that NF-κB activation may be involved. Angiotensinogen facilitates activation of angiotensin 2, an enzyme that is leaked into the airways as a result of increased vascular permeability during airway inflammation.[96] Genotypic variants in the angiotensinogen (*AGT*) gene (2401C>G and 2476C>T) could affect lung function abnormalities among patients with AERD[97] by modulating the angiotensin 2 enzyme, which can potentiate the effect of other bronchoconstrictor agents, such as the CysLTs. Angiotensin 1-converting enzyme (ACE) plays a pivotal role in the metabolism

**Table 1**
Predisposing genetic factors for aspirin hypersensitivity

| Group | Gene | Name | Genetic Variants | Phenotype | Year | References |
|---|---|---|---|---|---|---|
| I | ALOX5 | 5-lipoxygenase | SP-1 binding motif | AERD | 1997 | 8,15,16 |
| | COX-2 | Cyclooxygenase 2 | G-765C | AERD | 2004 | 23 |
| | CYSLTR1 | Cysteinyl leukotriene receptor1 | −634C>T, −475A>C, −336A>G | AERD | 2006 | 17 |
| | CYSLTR2 | Cysteinyl leukotriene receptor2 | −819T>C | AERD | 2005 | 20 |
| | LTC4S | Leukotriene C4 synthase | −444A>C | AERD | 1997 | 9 |
| | LTC4S | Leukotriene C4 synthase | −444A>C | AIU | 2004 | 39,40 |
| | PTGER | Prostaglandin E2 receptor | rs7543182 rs959 | AERD | 2007 | 28,29 |
| | EP2 | Prostaglandin E2 receptor | | AERD | 2004 | 24 |
| | TBXA2R | Thromboxane A2 receptor | +795T>C | AERD | 2005 | 32,33 |
| | TBXAS1 | Thromboxane A synthase | rs6962291 | AERD | 2011 | 31 |
| II | C6 | Complement 6 | rs10512766, rs4957374 | AERD | 2011 | 67 |
| | HLA | Human leukocyte antigen | DPB1*0301 | AERD | 2004 | 59,60 |
| | HLA | Human leukocyte antigen | DRB1*1302 | AIU | 2005 | 61 |
| | TAP2 | Transporter 1 and 2, ATP-binding cassette | Haplotype | AERD | 2011 | 68 |
| | TLR3 | Toll-like receptor 3 | −299698G>T and 293391G>A | AERD | 2011 | 75 |
| | UBE3C | Ubiquitin protein ligase E3C | rs10949635G>T | AERD | 2011 | 95 |
| | IL-10/TGF | Interleukin 10/transforming growth factor | −1082 A>G and −509C>T | AERD | 2009 | 113 |
| III | EMID2 | Emilin/multimerin domain-containing protein 2 | EMID2_BL2_ht2 | AERD | 2011 | 77 |
| | KIF3A | Kinesin family number 3A | rs 3756775 | AERD | 2011 | 82 |
| | SPINK5 | Serine protease inhibitor, Kazal type 5 | G1258A, A1103G | AERD | 2012 | 78 |

| | Gene | Gene name | Polymorphism | | Year | Ref |
|---|---|---|---|---|---|---|
| IV | ACE | Angiotensin converting enzyme | −262A>T, −115T>C | AERD | 2008 | 100 |
| | ADORA3 | Adenosine receptor | 1050G/T | AIU | 2010 | 108 |
| | AGT | Angiotensinogen | p2401C>G and p2476C>T | AERD | 2011 | 97 |
| | CACN6 | Calcium channel, voltage-dependent, gamma subunit 6 | rs192808C > T | AERD | 2010 | 88 |
| | PPARG | Peroxisome proliferator-activated receptors | 82466C>T (His449His) | AERD | 2009 | 85 |
| | SLC5A12 | Betaine/GABA member 12 | rs557881 | AERD | 2010 | 86 |
| | STK10 | Serine/threonine kinase 10 | rs2306961 | AERD | 2011 | 93 |
| V | CCF3 | Chemokine, CC motif, receptor 3 | −520T>C | AERD | 2010 | 51 |
| | CRTH2 | Prostaglandin D2 receptor | −466T>C | AERD | 2010 | 52 |
| | IL-13 | Interleukin 13 | 1510A>C,1055C>T, Arg110Gln | AERD | 2010 | 50 |
| | IL-4 | Interleukin 4 | −589T C and −33 C alleles | AERD | 2010 | 53 |
| | FcεRIα | Alpha chain of high-affinity IgE receptor I | −344C>T | AIU | 2007 | 54 |
| | HNMT | Histamine N-methyl transferase | 939A>G | AIU | 2009 | 55 |
| | IL-18 | Interleukin-18 | 607A>C, 137 G>C | AIU | 2011 | 57 |
| VI | CYP2C19 | Cytochrome P450 2C19 | 681G>A, 636G>A | AERD | 2011 | 110 |
| | CYP2C9 | Cytochrome P450 2C9 | −1188T>C | AIU | 2012 | 108 |
| | NAT2 | N-acetyltransferase | −9246G>C | AERD | 2010 | 109 |

I. Dysregulation of arachidonic acid metabolism. II. Initiation of immune response. III. Dysfunction of epithelial cells. IV. Biochemical signaling pathways in inflammatory cells. V. Effector function of inflammatory cells. VI. Aspirin metabolism.

of peptides including kinins and substance-P, which are involved in the pathogenesis of asthma.[98] Inhibition of ACE may lead to bronchial hyperreactivity.[99] The promoter polymorphism of the *ACE* gene (-262 A>T) may confer aspirin hypersensitivity in asthmatics by down-regulating *ACE* gene expression.[100] This finding suggests that decreased ACE activity may enhance airway inflammation and hyper-reactivity against aspirin hypersensitivity via endogenous peptides.[100]

Adenosine may contribute to aspirin hypersensitivity by interfering with oxidative phosphorylation leading to ATP catabolism[101] and adenosine deaminase inhibition.[102] These changes ultimately result in adenosine accumulation, which has diverse effects on cells, such as inducing bronchoconstriction in asthmatics,[103] altering airway inflammation, and modulating inflammatory mediators from mast cells.[104–106] A genetic study on AIU in a Korean population suggested a significant association between the adenosine A3 receptor (*ADORA3*) promoter polymorphism at -1050 G/T and the AIU phenotype due to the modulation of transcriptional activity and enhancement basophil histamine release from human mast cells.[107]

Overall, these findings provide evidence that non-COX target molecules of aspirin and/or NSAIDs involved in the inflammatory cell biochemical pathways may concomitantly contribute to the genetic predisposition to aspirin hypersensitivity.

### Aspirin Metabolism

The metabolic pathways of drug inactivation and elimination, in case of NSAIDs through oxidation by cytochrome P450 (CYP), glucuronide conjugation by UDP-glucuronosyltransferase (UGT), sulfate conjugation (sulfotransferases), and acetylation by *N*-acetyltransferase (NAT), may be involved in aspirin hypersensitivity. Specifically, interindividual differences in the metabolizing activities of these enzymes may be the underlying cause of aspirin hypersensitivity. Among the metabolizing enzymes, *CYP2C9, NAT2,* and *UGT1A6* gene polymorphisms have been investigated in aspirin hypersensitivity. As a result, the C allele of *CYP2C9* −1188T>C is significantly associated with the AIU phenotype,[108] whereas the genetic variants of the *NAT2* (-9246G>C) and *CYP2C19* (681G>A, 636G>A) genes are significantly associated with the AERD phenotype.[109,110] However, functional effects of these polymorphisms have not been examined. The *NAT* gene polymorphism can also affect proinflammatory CysLTs by their inactivation through *N*-acetylation.[111,112]

## LIMITATION OF CURRENT GENETIC STUDIES AND FUTURE PERSPECTIVES

Despite recent advances in genetic studies on aspirin hypersensitivity, the genetic mechanisms underlying aspirin hypersensitivity are not fully understood. The multifactorial etiology of aspirin hypersensitivity may be 1 of the reasons, likewise polygenetic effects documented by association studies. Genetic contributions can be modulated by interaction with environmental factors, and multiple genetic interactions may synergistically contribute to the aspirin hypersensitivity phenotype.

### Gene–Gene Interactions

A few studies have shown synergistic gene–gene interactions in the genetic mechanism of AERD. Gene–gene interactions between the TGFβ1-509C/T and IL-10-1082A/G polymorphisms have been addressed in patients with AERD and chronic rhinosinusitis.[113] Moreoever, Kim and colleagues[114] reported a 4-locus genetic interaction in the susceptibility to aspirin intolerance in patients with asthma. Out of all the multifactor dimensionality reduction models analyzed, one 4-locus model, consisting of the *B2ADR (β2 adrenergic receptor)* 46A>G, *CCR3*–520T>G, *CysLTR1*–634C>T, and *FCER1B* −109T>C showed the highest diagnostic values. These findings suggest that a multilocus SNP set can be applied to predict the genetic susceptibility to AERD.

Until now, despite intensive genetic studies using the candidate gene approach and more recently using GWAS, most genetic polymorphisms identified as risk factors have had an odds ratio of less than 2, indicating that genetic polymorphisms contribute to susceptibility, but their effects may be smaller than expected. Therefore, other parallel approaches should be considered.

### Epigenetics

Epigenetic modification including DNA methylation, histone modification, and gene silencing by micro-RNA could silence (loss of function) or activate (gain of function) genes by controlling gene expression in response to biologic or environmental changes. An environmental epigenetic investigation of AERD has been reported.[115] Comparing the entire methylation profile of nasal polyps from patients with AERD and aspirin-tolerant asthma, differences in methylation levels of several hundred genes were found. In particular, among the arachidonate pathway genes, PGE synthase was hypermethylated, and PGD synthase, arachidonate 5-lipoxygenase activating protein, leukotriene B4 receptor, and the lipoxygenase homology domain 1 were hypomethylated, which suggested that different methylation patterns may be responsible for the AERD phenotype. Therefore, further epigenetic studies will provide novel information regarding the gene–environment interaction.

### Next-Generation Sequencing

The currently used SNP genotyping platforms mostly target common sequence variants with greater than 5% minor allele frequency. Therefore, genome wide sequencing may be required to obtain more information on rare variants that may confer genetic susceptibility to aspirin. Whole-genome sequencing or exome sequencing may be useful to detect rare variants involved in the pathogenesis of aspirin hypersensitivity. The full genome sequencing project of 1000 anonymous subjects, known as the 1000 Genomes Project (http://www.1000genomes.org/page.php), has commenced, and the cost of whole genome sequencing has been decreasing rapidly. Therefore, next-generation sequencing technology can be applied to genetic studies on aspirin hypersensitivity in the near future.

## SUMMARY

Based on genetic association studies, it has been learned that persistent inflammation with marked inflammatory cell activation, unbalanced leukotrien production, complement activation, and enhanced biochemical signaling cascades may be important pathogenic mechanisms underlying aspirin hypersensitivity and that several genetic polymorphisms may be involved. However, one should also consider epigenetic factors, heterogeneous inflammatory cells, and interindividual variability in drug metabolism combined with variations in immunologic backgrounds as underlying mechanisms. Further, extensive biologic and/or functional studies should be performed for a further comprehensive understanding of the complex etiology of aspirin hypersensitivity.

## REFERENCES

1. Szczeklik A, Stevenson DD. Aspirin-induced asthma: advances in pathogenesis, diagnosis, and management. J Allergy Clin Immunol 2003;111:913–21 [quiz: 922].

2. Stevenson DD, Sanchez-Borges M, Szczeklik A. Classification of allergic and pseudoallergic reactions to drugs that inhibit cyclooxygenase enzymes. Ann Allergy Asthma Immunol 2001;87:177–80.

3. Grattan CE. Aspirin sensitivity and urticaria. Clin Exp Dermatol 2003;28:123–7.

4. Kowalski ML, Makowska JS, Blanca M, et al. Hypersensitivity to nonsteroidal anti-inflammatory drugs (NSAIDs) - classification, diagnosis and management: review of the EAACI/ENDA(#) and GA2LEN/HANNA*. Allergy 2011;66:818–29.

5. Szczeklik A. The cyclooxygenase theory of aspirin-induced asthma. Eur Respir J 1990;3:588–93.

6. Celik G, Bavbek S, Misirligil Z, et al. Release of cysteinyl leukotrienes with aspirin stimulation and the effect of prostaglandin E(2) on this release from peripheral blood leucocytes in aspirin-induced asthmatic patients. Clin Exp Allergy 2001;31:1615–22.

7. Kowalski ML, Pawliczak R, Wozniak J, et al. Differential metabolism of arachidonic acid in nasal polyp epithelial cells cultured from aspirin-sensitive and aspirin-tolerant patients. Am J Respir Crit Care Med 2000;161:391–8.

8. In KH, Asano K, Beier D, et al. Naturally occurring mutations in the human 5-lipoxygenase gene promoter that modify transcription factor binding and reporter gene transcription. J Clin Invest 1997;99:1130–7.

9. Sanak M, Simon HU, Szczeklik A. Leukotriene C4 synthase promoter polymorphism and risk of aspirin-induced asthma. Lancet 1997;350:1599–600.

10. Peters-Golden M, Henderson WR Jr. Leukotrienes. N Engl J Med 2007;357: 1841–54.

11. Sanak M, Pierzchalska M, Bazan-Socha S, et al. Enhanced expression of the leukotriene C(4) synthase due to overactive transcription of an allelic variant associated with aspirin-intolerant asthma. Am J Respir Cell Mol Biol 2000;23: 290–6.

12. Cowburn AS, Sladek K, Soja J, et al. Overexpression of leukotriene C4 synthase in bronchial biopsies from patients with aspirin-intolerant asthma. J Clin Invest 1998;101:834–46.

13. Cai Y, Bjermer L, Halstensen TS. Bronchial mast cells are the dominating LTC4S-expressing cells in aspirin-tolerant asthma. Am J Respir Cell Mol Biol 2003;29: 683–93.

14. Adamjee J, Suh YJ, Park HS, et al. Expression of 5-lipoxygenase and cyclooxygenase pathway enzymes in nasal polyps of patients with aspirin-intolerant asthma. J Pathol 2006;209:392–9.

15. Kim SH, Bae JS, Suh CH, et al. Polymorphism of tandem repeat in promoter of 5-lipoxygenase in ASA-intolerant asthma: a positive association with airway hyperresponsiveness. Allergy 2005;60:760–5.

16. Drazen JM. Pharmacology of leukotriene receptor antagonists and 5-lipoxygenase inhibitors in the management of asthma. Pharmacotherapy 1997;17: 22S–30S.

17. Kim SH, Oh JM, Kim YS, et al. Cysteinyl leukotriene receptor 1 promoter polymorphism is associated with aspirin-intolerant asthma in males. Clin Exp Allergy 2006;36:433–9.

18. Sousa AR, Parikh A, Scadding G, et al. Leukotriene-receptor expression on nasal mucosal inflammatory cells in aspirin-sensitive rhinosinusitis. N Engl J Med 2002;347:1493–9.

19. Kim SH, Ye YM, Hur GY, et al. CysLTR1 promoter polymorphism and requirement for leukotriene receptor antagonist in aspirin-intolerant asthma patients. Pharmacogenomics 2007;8:1143–50.

20. Park JS, Chang HS, Park CS, et al. Association analysis of cysteinyl-leukotriene receptor 2 (CYSLTR2) polymorphisms with aspirin intolerance in asthmatics. Pharmacogenet Genomics 2005;15:483–92.
21. Farooque SP, Lee TH. Aspirin-sensitive respiratory disease. Annu Rev Physiol 2009;71:465–87.
22. Ciana P, Fumagalli M, Trincavelli ML, et al. The orphan receptor GPR17 identified as a new dual uracil nucleotides/cysteinyl-leukotrienes receptor. EMBO J 2006;25:4615–27.
23. Szczeklik W, Sanak M, Szczeklik A. Functional effects and gender association of COX-2 gene polymorphism G-765C in bronchial asthma. J Allergy Clin Immunol 2004;114:248–53.
24. Jinnai N, Sakagami T, Sekigawa T, et al. Polymorphisms in the prostaglandin E2 receptor subtype 2 gene confer susceptibility to aspirin-intolerant asthma: a candidate gene approach. Hum Mol Genet 2004;13:3203–17.
25. Picado C, Fernandez-Morata JC, Juan M, et al. Cyclooxygenase-2 mRNA is downexpressed in nasal polyps from aspirin-sensitive asthmatics. Am J Respir Crit Care Med 1999;160:291–6.
26. Coleman RA, Smith WL, Narumiya S. International Union of Pharmacology classification of prostanoid receptors: properties, distribution, and structure of the receptors and their subtypes. Pharmacol Rev 1994;46:205–29.
27. Narumiya S, Sugimoto Y, Ushikubi F. Prostanoid receptors: structures, properties, and functions. Physiol Rev 1999;79:1193–226.
28. Kim SH, Kim YK, Park HW, et al. Association between polymorphisms in prostanoid receptor genes and aspirin-intolerant asthma. Pharmacogenet Genomics 2007;17:295–304.
29. Park BL, Park SM, Park JS, et al. Association of PTGER gene family polymorphisms with aspirin intolerant asthma in Korean asthmatics. BMB Rep 2010; 43:445–9.
30. Needleman P, Turk J, Jakschik BA, et al. Arachidonic acid metabolism. Annu Rev Biochem 1986;55:69–102.
31. Oh SH, Kim YH, Park SM, et al. Association analysis of thromboxane A synthase 1 gene polymorphisms with aspirin intolerance in asthmatic patients. Pharmacogenomics 2011;12:351 63.
32. Kim SH, Choi JH, Park HS, et al. Association of thromboxane A2 receptor gene polymorphism with the phenotype of acetyl salicylic acid-intolerant asthma. Clin Exp Allergy 2005;35:585–90.
33. Kohyama K, Hashimoto M, Abe S, et al. Thromboxane A2 receptor +795T>C and chemoattractant receptor-homologous molecule expressed on Th2 cells -466T>C gene polymorphisms in patients with aspirin-exacerbated respiratory disease. Mol Med Report 2012;5:477–82.
34. Kowalski ML, Ptasinska A, Jedrzejczak M, et al. Aspirin-triggered 15-HETE generation in peripheral blood leukocytes is a specific and sensitive Aspirin-Sensitive Patients Identification Test (ASPITest). Allergy 2005;60:1139–45.
35. Song YS, Yang EM, Kim SH, et al. Effect of genetic polymorphism of ALOX15 on aspirin-exacerbated respiratory disease. Int Arch Allergy Immunol 2012;159: 157–61.
36. McMahon B, Godson C. Lipoxins: endogenous regulators of inflammation. Am J Physiol Renal Physiol 2004;286:F189–201.
37. Kim HJ, Cho SH, Park JS, et al. Association analysis of formyl peptide receptor 2 (FPR2) polymorphisms and Aspirin exacerbated respiratory diseases. J Hum Genet 2012;57:247–53.

38. Feltenmark S, Gautam N, Brunnstrom A, et al. Eoxins are proinflammatory arachidonic acid metabolites produced via the 15-lipoxygenase-1 pathway in human eosinophils and mast cells. Proc Natl Acad Sci U S A 2008;105: 680–5.

39. Mastalerz L, Setkowicz M, Szczeklik A. Mechanism of chronic urticaria exacerbation by aspirin. Curr Allergy Asthma Rep 2005;5:277–83.

40. Mastalerz L, Setkowicz M, Sanak M, et al. Hypersensitivity to aspirin: common eicosanoid alterations in urticaria and asthma. J Allergy Clin Immunol 2004; 113:771–5.

41. Mastalerz L, Setkowicz M, Sanak M, et al. Familial aggregation of aspirin-induced urticaria and leukotriene C synthase allelic variant. Br J Dermatol 2006;154:256–60.

42. Kim SH, Yang EM, Park HJ, et al. Differential contribution of the CysLTR1 gene in patients with aspirin hypersensitivity. J Clin Immunol 2007;27:613–9.

43. Higashi N, Taniguchi M, Mita H, et al. Clinical features of asthmatic patients with increased urinary leukotriene E4 excretion (hyperleukotrienuria): involvement of chronic hyperplastic rhinosinusitis with nasal polyposis. J Allergy Clin Immunol 2004;113:277–83.

44. Antczak A, Montuschi P, Kharitonov S, et al. Increased exhaled cysteinyl-leukotrienes and 8-isoprostane in aspirin-induced asthma. Am J Respir Crit Care Med 2002;166:301–6.

45. Szczeklik A, Sladek K, Dworski R, et al. Bronchial aspirin challenge causes specific eicosanoid response in aspirin-sensitive asthmatics. Am J Respir Crit Care Med 1996;154:1608–14.

46. Fischer AR, Rosenberg MA, Lilly CM, et al. Direct evidence for a role of the mast cell in the nasal response to aspirin in aspirin-sensitive asthma. J Allergy Clin Immunol 1994;94:1046–56.

47. Sousa A, Pfister R, Christie PE, et al. Enhanced expression of cyclo-oxygenase isoenzyme 2 (COX-2) in asthmatic airways and its cellular distribution in aspirin-sensitive asthma. Thorax 1997;52:940–5.

48. Varga EM, Jacobson MR, Masuyama K, et al. Inflammatory cell populations and cytokine mRNA expression in the nasal mucosa in aspirin-sensitive rhinitis. Eur Respir J 1999;14:610–5.

49. Nasser SM, Pfister R, Christie PE, et al. Inflammatory cell populations in bronchial biopsies from aspirin-sensitive asthmatic subjects. Am J Respir Crit Care Med 1996;153:90–6.

50. Palikhe NS, Kim SH, Cho BY, et al. IL-13 gene polymorphisms are associated with rhinosinusitis and eosinophilic inflammation in aspirin intolerant asthma. Allergy Asthma Immunol Res 2010;2:134–40.

51. Kim SH, Yang EM, Lee HN, et al. Association of the CCR3 gene polymorphism with aspirin exacerbated respiratory disease. Respir Med 2010;104: 626–32.

52. Palikhe NS, Kim SH, Cho BY, et al. Genetic variability in CRTH2 polymorphism increases eotaxin-2 levels in patients with aspirin exacerbated respiratory disease. Allergy 2010;65:338–46.

53. Kim BS, Park SM, Uhm TG, et al. Effect of single nucleotide polymorphisms within the interleukin-4 promoter on aspirin intolerance in asthmatics and interleukin-4 promoter activity. Pharmacogenet Genomics 2010;20:748–58.

54. Bae JS, Kim SH, Ye YM, et al. Significant association of FcεRIα promoter polymorphisms with aspirin-intolerant chronic urticaria. J Allergy Clin Immunol 2007; 119:449–56.

55. Kim SH, Kang YM, Cho BY, et al. Histamine N-methyltransferase 939A>G poly-morphism affects mRNA stability in patients with acetylsalicylic acid-intolerant chronic urticaria. Allergy 2009;64:213–21.
56. Laidlaw TM, Kidder MS, Bhattacharyya N, et al. Cysteinyl leukotriene overpro-duction in aspirin-exacerbated respiratory disease is driven by platelet-adherent leukocytes. Blood 2012;119:3790–8.
57. Choi SJ, Ye YM, Hur GY, et al. Neutrophil activation in patients with ASA-induced urticaria. J Clin Immunol 2008;28:244–9.
58. Kim SH, Son JK, Yang EM, et al. A functional promoter polymorphism of the human IL-18 gene is associated with aspirin-induced urticaria. Br J Dermatol 2011;165:976–84.
59. Choi JH, Lee KW, Oh HB, et al. HLA association in aspirin-intolerant asthma: DPB1*0301 as a strong marker in a Korean population. J Allergy Clin Immunol 2004;113:562–4.
60. Park HS, Kim SH, Sampson AP, et al. The HLA-DPB1*0301 marker might predict the requirement for leukotriene receptor antagonist in patients with aspirin-intolerant asthma. J Allergy Clin Immunol 2004;114:688–9.
61. Kim SH, Choi JH, Lee KW, et al. The human leucocyte antigen-DRB1*1302-DQB1*0609-DPB1*0201 haplotype may be a strong genetic marker for aspirin-induced urticaria. Clin Exp Allergy 2005;35:339–44.
62. Moffatt MF, Kabesch M, Liang L, et al. Genetic variants regulating ORMDL3 expression contribute to the risk of childhood asthma. Nature 2007;448: 470–3.
63. Himes BE, Hunninghake GM, Baurley JW, et al. Genome-wide association anal-ysis identifies PDE4D as an asthma-susceptibility gene. Am J Hum Genet 2009; 84:581–93.
64. Li X, Howard TD, Zheng SL, et al. Genome-wide association study of asthma identifies RAD50-IL13 and HLA-DR/DQ regions. J Allergy Clin Immunol 2010; 125:328–335.e311.
65. Gudbjartsson DF, Bjornsdottir US, Halapi E, et al. Sequence variants affecting eosinophil numbers associate with asthma and myocardial infarction. Nat Genet 2009;41:342–7.
66. Kim JH, Park BL, Cheong HS, et al. Genome-wide and follow-up studies identify CEP68 gene variants associated with risk of aspirin-intolerant asthma. PLoS One 2010;5:e13818.
67. Kim SH, Ye YM, Palikhe NS, et al. Genetic and ethnic risk factors associated with drug hypersensitivity. Curr Opin Allergy Clin Immunol 2010;10:280–90.
68. Kim JH, Park BL, Pasaje CF, et al. Genetic association analysis of TAP1 and TAP2 polymorphisms with aspirin exacerbated respiratory disease and its FEV1 decline. J Hum Genet 2011;56:652–9.
69. Babu KS, Salvi SS. Aspirin and asthma. Chest 2000;118:1470–6.
70. Lee SH, Rhim T, Choi YS, et al. Complement C3a and C4a increased in plasma of patients with aspirin-induced asthma. Am J Respir Crit Care Med 2006;173: 370–8.
71. Pasaje CF, Bae JS, Park BL, et al. Association analysis of C6 genetic variations and aspirin hypersensitivity in Korean asthmatic patients. Hum Immunol 2011; 72:973–8.
72. Szczeklik A. Aspirin-induced asthma as a viral disease. Clin Allergy 1988;18: 15–20.
73. Filipowicz E, Sanak M. Exacerbation of aspirin-induced asthma associated with RSV infection. Przegl Lek 2003;60:185–7 [in Polish].

74. Yoshida S, Sakamoto H, Yamawaki Y, et al. Effect of acyclovir on bronchocon-striction and urinary leukotriene E4 excretion in aspirin-induced asthma. J Allergy Clin Immunol 1998;102:909–14.
75. Palikhe NS, Kim SH, Kim JH, et al. Role of toll-like receptor 3 variants in aspirin-exacerbated respiratory disease. Allergy Asthma Immunol Res 2011;3:123–7.
76. Polito AJ, Proud D. Epithelia cells as regulators of airway inflammation. J Allergy Clin Immunol 1998;102:714–8.
77. Pasaje CF, Kim JH, Park BL, et al. A possible association of EMID2 polymor-phisms with aspirin hypersensitivity in asthma. Immunogenetics 2011;63:13–21.
78. Fruth K, Goebel G, Koutsimpelas D, et al. Low SPINK5 expression in chronic rhi-nosinusitis. Laryngoscope 2012;122:1198–204.
79. Bush A, Cole P, Hariri M, et al. Primary ciliary dyskinesia: diagnosis and stan-dards of care. Eur Respir J 1998;12:982–8.
80. Marszalek JR, Ruiz-Lozano P, Roberts E, et al. Situs inversus and embryonic ciliary morphogenesis defects in mouse mutants lacking the KIF3A subunit of kinesin-II. Proc Natl Acad Sci U S A 1999;96:5043–8.
81. Corbit KC, Shyer AE, Dowdle WE, et al. Kif3a constrains beta-catenin-dependent Wnt signaling through dual ciliary and non-ciliary mechanisms. Nat Cell Biol 2008;10:70–6.
82. Kim JH, Cha JY, Cheong HS, et al. KIF3A, a cilia structural gene on chromosome 5q31, and its polymorphisms show an association with aspirin hypersensitivity in asthma. J Clin Immunol 2011;31:112–21.
83. Kopp E, Ghosh S. Inhibition of NF-kappa B by sodium salicylate and aspirin. Science 1994;265:956–9.
84. Perez GM, Melo M, Keegan AD, et al. Aspirin and salicylates inhibit the IL-4- and IL-13-induced activation of STAT6. J Immunol 2002;168:1428–34.
85. Oh SH, Park SM, Park JS, et al. Association analysis of peroxisome proliferator-activated receptors gamma gene polymorphisms with asprin hypersensitivity in asthmatics. Allergy Asthma Immunol Res 2009;1:30–5.
86. Pasaje CF, Kim JH, Park BL, et al. Association of SLC6A12 variants with aspirin-intolerant asthma in a Korean population. Ann Hum Genet 2010;74:326–34.
87. Kim JY, Kim JH, Park TJ, et al. Positive association between aspirin-intolerant asthma and genetic polymorphisms of FSIP1: a case–case study. BMC Pulm Med 2010;10:34.
88. Lee JS, Kim JH, Bae JS, et al. Association of CACNG6 polymorphisms with aspirin-intolerance asthmatics in a Korean population. BMC Med Genet 2010; 11:138.
89. Benayoun L, Letuve S, Druilhe A, et al. Regulation of peroxisome proliferator-activated receptor gamma expression in human asthmatic airways: relationship with proliferation, apoptosis, and airway remodeling. Am J Respir Crit Care Med 2001;164:1487–94.
90. Xiang YY, Wang S, Liu M, et al. A GABAergic system in airway epithelium is essential for mucus overproduction in asthma. Nat Med 2007;13:862–7.
91. Wong WS, Leong KP. Tyrosine kinase inhibitors: a new approach for asthma. Biochim Biophys Acta 2004;1697:53–69.
92. Kumano K, Nakao A, Nakajima H, et al. Blockade of JAK2 by tyrphostin AG-490 inhibits antigen-induced eosinophil recruitment into the mouse airways. Bio-chem Biophys Res Commun 2000;270:209–14.
93. Kim JH, Park BL, Cheong HS, et al. Variations in the STK10 gene and possible associations with aspirin-intolerant asthma in a Korean population. J Investig Allergol Clin Immunol 2011;21:378–88.

94. Lee JS, Kim JH, Bae JS, et al. Association analysis of UBE3C polymorphisms in Korean aspirin-intolerant asthmatic patients. Ann Allergy Asthma Immunol 2010; 105:307–12.

95. Pasaje CF, Kim JH, Park BL, et al. UBE3C genetic variations as potent markers of nasal polyps in Korean asthma patients. J Hum Genet 2011;56:797–800.

96. Kanazawa H, Kurihara N, Hirata K, et al. Angiotensin II stimulates peptide leuko-triene production by guinea pig airway via the AT1 receptor pathway. Prosta-glandins Leukot Essent Fatty Acids 1995;52:241–4.

97. Pasaje CF, Kim JH, Park BL, et al. Association of the variants in AGT gene with modified drug response in Korean aspirin-intolerant asthma patients. Pulm Phar-macol Ther 2011;24:595–601.

98. Erdos EG. Angiotensin I converting enzyme and the changes in our concepts through the years. Lewis K. Dahl memorial lecture. Hypertension 1990;16: 363–70.

99. Bucknall CE, Neilly JB, Carter R, et al. Bronchial hyper-reactivity in patients who cough after receiving angiotensin converting enzyme inhibitors. Br Med J (Clin Res Ed) 1988;296:86–8.

100. Kim TH, Chang HS, Park SM, et al. Association of angiotensin I-converting enzyme gene polymorphisms with aspirin intolerance in asthmatics. Clin Exp Allergy 2008;38:1727–37.

101. Mingatto FE, Santos AC, Uyemura SA, et al. In vitro interaction of nonsteroidal anti-inflammatory drugs on oxidative phosphorylation of rat kidney mitochon-dria: respiration and ATP synthesis. Arch Biochem Biophys 1996;334:303–8.

102. Kopff A, Kopff M, Kowalczyk E. The influence of nonsteroidal anti-inflammatory drugs on deaminase adenosine activity. Pol Arch Med Wewn 2006;116:832–7 [in Polish].

103. Mann JS, Holgate ST, Renwick AG, et al. Airway effects of purine nucleosides and nucleotides and release with bronchial provocation in asthma. J Appl Phys-iol 1986;61:1667–76.

104. Peachell PT, Lichtenstein LM, Schleimer RP. Differential regulation of human basophil and lung mast cell function by adenosine. J Pharmacol Exp Ther 1991;256:717–26.

105. Forsythe P, Ennis M. Adenosine, mast cells and asthma. Inflamm Res 1999;48: 301–7.

106. Tilley SL, Wagoner VA, Salvatore CA, et al. Adenosine and inosine increase cutaneous vasopermeability by activating A(3) receptors on mast cells. J Clin Invest 2000;105:361–7.

107. Kim SH, Nam EJ, Kim YK, et al. Functional variability of the adenosine A3 receptor (ADORA3) gene polymorphism in aspirin-induced urticaria. Br J Der-matol 2010;163:977–85.

108. Palikhe NS, Kim SH, Nam YH, et al. Polymorphisms of aspirin-metabolizing enzymes CYP2C9, NAT2 and UGT1A6 in aspirin-intolerant urticaria. Allergy Asthma Immunol Res 2011;3:273–6.

109. Kim JM, Park BL, Park SM, et al. Association analysis of N-acetyl transferase-2 polymorphisms with aspirin intolerance among asthmatics. Pharmacogenomics 2010;11:951–0.

110. Kohyama K, Abe S, Kodaira K, et al. Polymorphisms of the CYP2C19 gene in Japanese patients with aspirin-exacerbated respiratory disease. J Allergy Clin Immunol 2011;128:1117–20.

111. Orning L. Omega-oxidation of cysteine-containing leukotrienes by rat-liver micro-somes. Isolation and characterization of omega-hydroxy and omega-carboxy

metabolites of leukotriene E4 and N-acetylleukotriene E4. Eur J Biochem 1987; 170:77–85.

112. Sala A, Voelkel N, Maclouf J, et al. Leukotriene E4 elimination and metabolism in normal human subjects. J Biol Chem 1990;265:21771–8.

113. Kim SH, Yang EM, Lee HN, et al. Combined effect of IL-10 and TGF-beta1 promoter polymorphisms as a risk factor for aspirin-intolerant asthma and rhinosinusitis. Allergy 2009;64:1221–5.

114. Kim SH, Jeong HH, Cho BY, et al. Association of four-locus gene interaction with aspirin-intolerant asthma in Korean asthmatics. J Clin Immunol 2008;28:336–42.

115. Cheong HS, Park SM, Kim MO, et al. Genome-wide methylation profile of nasal polyps: relation to aspirin hypersensitivity in asthmatics. Allergy 2011;66: 637–44.

# Pathogenesis of Aspirin-Exacerbated Respiratory Disease and Reactions

Tanya M. Laidlaw, MD, Joshua A. Boyce, MD*

## KEYWORDS

- Cysteinyl leukotriene • Cyclooxygenase • Prostaglandin $E_2$ • Thromboxane
- Eosinophil • Mast cell • Platelet • AERD

## KEY POINTS

- Pathogenesis of aspirin-exacerbated respiratory disease (AERD) involves a consistent pattern of aberrant leukotriene generation.
- AERD is associated with deregulated expression and function of enzymes and receptors responsible for the production and function of lipid mediators that are protective against reactions to cyclooxygenase inhibitors.
- AERD is acquired rather than hereditary.

## INTRODUCTION

Aspirin-exacerbated respiratory disease (AERD) is characterized by the quatrad of asthma, eosinophilic rhinosinusitis, nasal polyposis, and the onset of respiratory reactions after ingestion of aspirin or any other inhibitor of the cyclooxygenase 1 (COX-1) enzyme. Although precipitation of acute reactions by ingestion of COX-1 inhibitors is the defining feature of the syndrome, the underlying inflammatory respiratory disease process begins and continues independently of exposure to aspirin or nonsteroidal antiinflammatory drugs (NSAIDs). The clinical course of the respiratory disease is often stereotypical, which suggests a common underlying cause and mechanism. Typically, the syndrome begins with severe nasal congestion, often after an apparent viral upper respiratory infection in young adulthood, which progresses to chronic eosinophilic rhinosinusitis and recurrent nasal polyposis. During the evolution of the sinus disease, symptoms of lower respiratory tract disease also begin and persistent asthma is diagnosed. The asthma tends to be severe, and individuals with AERD have significantly

Brigham and Women's Hospital, Department of Medicine, Division of Rheumatology, Immunology and Allergy, Jeff and Penny Vinik Center for Allergic Disease Research, 75 Francis Street, Boston, MA 02115, USA
* Corresponding author.
E-mail address: jboyce@partners.org

Immunol Allergy Clin N Am 33 (2013) 195–210
http://dx.doi.org/10.1016/j.iac.2012.11.006
0889-8561/13/$ – see front matter © 2013 Elsevier Inc. All rights reserved.

immunology.theclinics.com

lower baseline lung function measurements than do those with aspirin-tolerant asthma, suggesting the effects of airway remodeling.[1] If patients with AERD ingest aspirin or an NSAID, an acute reaction develops, characterized by both upper and lower respiratory symptoms. Neither the pathophysiology of the underlying disease nor the mechanisms of the reactions to NSAIDs are entirely understood. Both the baseline respiratory pathology of AERD and the clinical reactions to NSAIDs are accompanied by aberrant metabolism of arachidonic acid, the precursor of both leukotrienes (LTs) and prostaglandins (PGs). This article reviews potential casual mechanisms responsible for the underlying disease, the confirmatory reactions to COX-1-active drugs, and the disturbances and pathogenetic roles of the lipid mediator systems.

## PATHOGENESIS OF THE UNDERLYING RESPIRATORY DISEASE
### Histopathology, Cytokines, and Microbes

Histologically, AERD is characterized by intense inflammation in the upper and lower airways. The numbers of eosinophils identified in the mucosal and submucosal compartments of bronchial and nasal biopsies exceed the numbers found in biopsies from aspirin-tolerant asthmatic individuals by 2 to 3-fold.[2,3] Degranulated mast cells are frequent. Lavage fluids obtained from the nasal and bronchial tissues show both higher percentages of eosinophils and higher levels of eosinophil cationic protein, when compared with lavage fluids from aspirin-tolerant controls.[3–5] Thus, even without aspirin provocation, there is evidence for an active, ongoing inflammatory response dominated by eosinophils and mast cells in the respiratory tissue in AERD. This persistent inflammation likely contributes substantially to the recurrent development of severe nasal polyps,[6] with the soluble products of eosinophils and mast cells causing edema and fibroproliferation.[7]

The mechanism by which granulocytes are drawn into the respiratory tissues is not fully understood. In individuals with AERD, aspirin challenges are associated with a significant increase in serum levels of eotaxin-2, a potent and selective chemoattractant for eosinophils.[8] A recent study[9] showed a markedly increased frequency of leukocytes associated with platelets in the nasal polyp specimens of patients with AERD compared with polyps from aspirin-tolerant controls (**Fig. 1**). Moreover, the percentages of eosinophils, neutrophils, and monocytes with adherent platelets were several-fold higher in the blood of individuals with AERD than in the blood of aspirin-tolerant controls. The platelet-adherent subsets of each leukocyte type expressed higher expression of both $\beta_1$-integrins and $\beta_2$-integrins than did the corresponding nonadherent subset. These findings suggest that a platelet-dependent pathway may facilitate inflammation of the respiratory mucosa in AERD by priming leukocytes for entry into the inflamed tissues. Resident eosinophils in the nasal polyps store interleukin 5 (IL-5) and granulocyte-macrophage colony-stimulating factor (GM-CSF), both of which are viability sustaining factors for eosinophils.[10] Another study reported that both mast cells and eosinophils staining positively for IL-5, as well as mast cells staining for GM-CSF, were several-fold higher in bronchial biopsies from patients with AERD than from aspirin-tolerant individuals.[11] These studies suggest that resident cells of the innate immune system contribute substantially to generating the cytokines that drive eosinophilic inflammation in a self-perpetuating fashion.

Although the histopathology of AERD supports the importance of effector cells of the allergic response, individuals with AERD frequently lack skin test reactivity to allergens commonly associated with allergic asthma and rhinosinusitis.[1,12] On average, total IgE levels tend to be slightly increased in the serum of patients with AERD

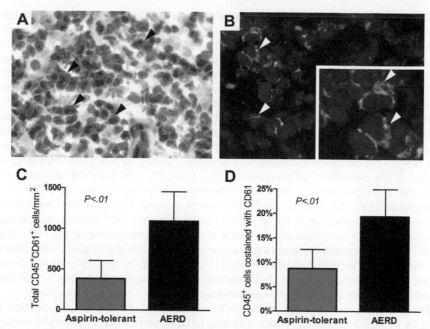

**Fig. 1.** Detection of platelet-leukocyte aggregates in nasal polyp tissue. (*A*) Hematoxylin-eosin staining of nasal polyp tissue from a patient with AERD shows many eosinophils (*black arrowheads*) and (*B*) immunofluorescent staining of the same tissue shows leukocytes (*green*, CD45$^+$) with adherent platelets (*red*, CD61$^+$) (*white arrowheads*). Photographs are shown at 400× magnification. (*C*) Total numbers of CD45$^+$ cells that colocalized with CD61 and (*D*) percentages of CD45$^+$ cells that colocalized with CD61 in the nasal polyp tissue from aspirin-tolerant controls with sinusitis (n = 4) and patients with AERD (n = 6). Data are expressed as mean + standard deviation. (*Data from* Laidlaw TM, Kidder MS, Bhattacharyya N, et al. Cysteinyl leukotriene overproduction in aspirin-exacerbated respiratory disease is driven by platelet-adherent leukocytes. Blood 2012;119:3790–98.)

compared with nonasthmatic controls, but lower than the levels found in the serum of atopic, aspirin-tolerant individuals[1,13] Some studies have identified higher levels of specific IgE against staphylococcal enterotoxin B in serum[13] and nasal polyps[14] from patients with AERD than from aspirin-tolerant controls. It is unclear whether these findings represent a direct causal relationship to staphylococcal colonization, or whether IgE responses to *Staphylococcus aureus* or its toxins reflect an upstream perturbation of an aberrant immune response to other microbes. Although a microbial pathogenesis has long been suspected in AERD, no consistent microbial isolates (including *Staphylococcus*) have been reported, nor are there geographic patterns suggestive of outbreaks.

## LIPID MEDIATORS IN THE PATHOGENESIS OF AERD
### Cysteinyl LTs

A fundamental characteristic of AERD is striking overproduction of cysteinyl LTs (cysLTs), a class of potent lipid inflammatory mediators derived from arachidonic acid.[15,16] Mast cells, eosinophils, and platelet-adherent leukocytes, all of which abound in the respiratory tissue of patients with AERD, each have the capacity to synthesize LTC$_4$, the parent cysLT, although it is unclear if the overproduction of cysLTs represents a fundamental abnormality or is a consequence of greater numbers and activation of these inflammatory cells. After liberation of arachidonic acid by cytosolic phospholipase $A_2$, arachidonic acid is oxidized by 5-lipoxygenase (LO) to form the unstable intermediate $LTA_4$, which is then conjugated to reduced glutathione by the terminal enzyme $LTC_4$ synthase ($LTC_4S$) to form $LTC_4$. $LTC_4$ is exported from the cell and enzymatically converted into $LTD_4$ and then into the stable end-metabolite $LTE_4$. Baseline urinary $LTE_4$ levels, a marker of systemic cysLT production, are 3 to 5 times higher in patients with AERD than in their aspirin-tolerant counterparts.[15] These levels increase further from the increased baseline (by as much as 10-fold) after challenges with COX-1-active drugs (see later discussion). Baseline levels of $LTE_4$ predict the magnitude of bronchoconstriction occurring during provocative aspirin challenges.[17] The short-lived LT mediators, $LTC_4$ and $LTD_4$, and their stable metabolite $LTE_4$ can all induce edema, bronchoconstriction, and airway mucous secretion.[18–20] In addition, $LTE_4$, the weakest bronchoconstrictor of the 3 cysLTs, induces marked recruitment of eosinophils to the airways in asthmatic patients.[21] Animal models also support a role for cysLTs in driving tissue fibrosis and airway remodeling.[22,23] Thus, cysLTs almost certainly contribute to the chronic inflammation and airway remodeling characteristic of AERD. The pathogenetic importance of the cysLTs in AERD is validated by the efficacy of drugs that interfere with their synthesis or block 1 of their receptors,[24,25] both of which improve disease control and sinonasal function.

There are several potential mechanistic explanations for the overproduction of cysLTs in AERD. Platelets, which express $LTC_4S$, can convert leukocyte-derived $LTA_4$ to $LTC_4$ when they adhere to 5-LO-expressing leukocytes.[26,27] Leukocyte-adherent platelets accounted for most $LTC_4S$ activity among peripheral blood granulocytes isolated from the blood of individuals with AERD, and the levels of urinary $LTE_4$ correlated strongly with the frequencies of platelet-adherent eosinophils, neutrophils, and monocytes.[9] Immunohistochemical studies indicated that eosinophils in bronchial and sinonasal biopsies from individuals with AERD show selective overexpression of $LTC_4S$ protein, but not 5-LO or 5-LO-activating protein.[3] Accordingly, peripheral blood eosinophils from individuals with AERD express more mRNA for *LTC4S* than do eosinophils from aspirin-tolerant controls.[28] A common polymorphic variant of the *LTC4S* allele shows a higher degree of promoter activity than the wild-type allele and was associated with an increased risk of AERD in a Polish population.[28] However, this association was not replicated in a cohort from the United States.[29] The percentages of mast cells and eosinophils in bronchial biopsies from patients with AERD staining positively for 5-LO were several-fold higher than in biopsies from aspirin-tolerant asthmatic controls.[30] Impaired functions of $PGE_2$, a COX pathway product that suppresses the activity of 5-LO (see later discussion), could also contribute to cysLT overproduction in AERD. Thus, overproduction of cysLTs likely relates to factors that both increase the activity of 5-LO and the availability of the substrate $LTA_4$, and increase the availability of the terminal enzyme, $LTC_4S$, including increased granulocyte-adherent platelets and increased $LTC_4S$ expression by eosinophils.

### CysLT Receptors

In addition to overproduction of cysLTs, individuals with AERD also show enhanced end-organ reactivity to the cysLTs. The functions of cysLTs are mediated by at least 2 G protein-coupled receptors (GPCRs), termed $CysLT_1R$ and $CysLT_2R$. The existence of yet-to-be-discovered cysLT receptors (CysLTRs) is likely, based on studies performed in receptor-null mice.[31,32] The high-affinity receptor for $LTD_4$, $CysLT_1R$, is overexpressed in nasal tissue inflammatory cells of patients with AERD compared with aspirin-tolerant controls.[33] The cause of this increased receptor expression is not known, although there are 3 single nucleotide polymorphisms (SNPs) in the promoter region of *CYSLTR1* in which mutant variants have been found to be associated with AERD. The mutant variants showed higher promoter activity, suggesting that these polymorphisms could modulate $CysLT_1R$ expression and lead to increased susceptibility to AERD.[34] Although $CysLT_1R$ has trivial affinity for $LTE_4$, patients with AERD show a selective hyperresponsiveness to bronchoconstriction induced by inhaled $LTE_4$ compared with aspirin-tolerant asthmatic controls,[35] suggesting that AERD involves additional upregulation of an unidentified $LTE_4$-specific receptor. Polymorphisms in the *CYSLTR2* gene encoding $CysLT_2R$, which negatively regulates the actions of $CysLT_1R$,[36,37] are also associated with AERD, and certain alleles were associated with the magnitude in the decrement in $FEV_1$ (forced expiratory volume in first second of expiration) measured during aspirin provocation.[38] Collectively, these observations suggest that the end-organ reactivity to cysLTs that characterizes AERD may be partly caused by genetically determined patterns of CysLTR expression or function. Moreover, the selective $LTE_4$ hyperresponsiveness in the face of high systemic levels is consistent with a potentially unique role for this stable end-metabolite of cysLTs in driving the disease.

## COX PATHWAY PRODUCTS IN AERD
### Proinflammatory PGs

PGs derive from COX-dependent metabolism of arachidonic acid. The COX-derived precursor, $PGH_2$, is converted to 1 of 5 bioactive terminal products ($PGE_2$, $PGF_2$, $PGI_2$, $PGD_2$, and thromboxane $A_2$ [$TXA_2$]) by corresponding isoform-specific synthases (**Fig. 2**). These terminal PG synthases show cell-selective expression and in some instances preferential coupling to COX-1, the more aspirin-sensitive COX

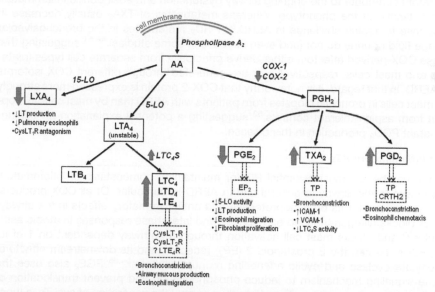

**Fig. 2.** Metabolism of arachidonic acid. Pathways of arachidonic acid metabolism involved in the pathogenesis of AERD. Enzymes are in italics, relevant receptors are in dashed boxes, and consequences of signaling through each receptor are in bulleted lists. Thick gray arrows show whether expression and function of each enzyme or product are increased or decreased in patients with AERD.

isoform, or to COX-2, which is more resistant to inhibition by aspirin.[39] Based on their pharmacologic properties, some PGs are candidate pathogenic effectors in AERD. $TXA_2$, the dominant COX product of platelets, which can also be generated by monocytes, mast cells, and granulocytes, is a potent bronchoconstrictor[40] and an inducer of endothelial adhesion molecule expression (intercellular adhesion molecule 1 [ICAM-1] and vascular cell adhesion molecule).[41] Metabolites of $TXA_2$ are present in higher levels in bronchoalveolar lavage fluid from patients with AERD compared with aspirin-tolerant asthmatics at baseline,[5] potentially reflecting the presence of platelets in the respiratory tissue (see **Fig. 1**). Furthermore, $TXA_2$ may be involved in the bronchoconstrictive effects of cysLTs, because the increase in airway resistance induced by either $LTC_4$ or $LTD_4$ in guinea pigs is prevented by a selective $TXA_2$ synthase inhibitor.[42] Moreover, the potentiation of histamine reactivity of human and guinea pig bronchi by $LTE_4$ could be blocked by an antagonist of the T prostanoid (TP) receptor, the only high-affinity receptor for $TXA_2$, or by pretreatment of the tissues with indomethacin to block COX function.[43] Thus, some of the clinical pharmacology of $LTE_4$ may relate to an incompletely explained capacity for this mediator to use $TXA_2$ or TP receptors as effectors. Although immunohistochemical studies of the TP receptor are lacking because of the lack of specific antibodies, there are 2 SNPs of the *TBXA2R* that are associated with AERD in a Korean population.[44]

$PGD_2$ is the dominant COX pathway product of mast cells.[45] Baseline levels of $PGD_2$ metabolites are higher in the serum and nasal polyps from patients with AERD than in samples from aspirin-tolerant controls,[46] possibly reflecting the ongoing activation of mast cells in AERD. $PGD_2$ is a bronchoconstrictor,[47] presumably through the effects of its stable metabolite, $9\alpha,11\beta$-$PGF_2$, acting at TP receptors.[48] $PGD_2$, acting through the CRTH2 receptor, is also a potent chemoattractant for eosinophils.[49] The persistent production of $PGD_2$ in the inflamed respiratory tissues of patients with AERD may therefore contribute to the ongoing airway dysfunction and eosinophilic inflammation characteristic of the phenotype. Whereas metabolites of $TXA_2$ usually decrease in response to aspirin challenge in AERD,[50] $PGD_2$ metabolites in the bronchoalveolar lavage fluid or urine do not (and even increase in some studies),[46,51] suggesting that these COX-derived effectors either derive principally from separate cell types (platelets and mast cells, respectively), or are generated through different COX isoforms in AERD. In that regard, it is noteworthy that COX-2 protein is expressed more strongly by mast cells in bronchial biopsies from patients with AERD than by mast cells in biopsies from aspirin-tolerant controls,[52] suggesting a potential explanation for aspirin-resistant $PGD_2$ production in this disease.

## Antiinflammatory PGs

$PGE_2$ may be the most essential PG for maintaining homeostasis of inflammatory responses in the airway in general and in AERD in particular. Of all COX products, $PGE_2$ is unique for its bronchoprotective and antiinflammatory effects in the airway. $PGE_2$ blocks allergen-induced early-phase and late-phase responses in atopic asthmatics[53] and blocks mast cell activation through a pathway dependent on 1 of its 4 GPCRs, termed the E prostanoid 2 ($EP_2$) receptor, and its downstream effectors, adenylate cyclase and cyclic adenosine monophosphate.[54,55] $PGE_2$ also uses the same signaling mechanism to induce phosphorylation and prevent translocation of 5-LO to the nuclear envelope[56] and can thus control the generation of cysLTs, a function that may be especially relevant to AERD. The importance of this potential mechanism is supported by the fact that inhaled $PGE_2$ prevents both the airway obstruction and the increase in urinary $LTE_4$ occurring in response to aspirin challenge in patients with AERD.[57] $PGE_2$ also potently inhibits eosinophil migration,[58] and both endogenous and exogenous $PGE_2$ suppress allergen-induced pulmonary eosinophil accumulation in humans[53] and rodents.[59] $PGE_2$ signals through $EP_2$ receptors to dampen the proliferation of fibroblasts and their production of collagen.[60] Collectively, these observations suggest that deficient $PGE_2$ generation or $EP_2$ receptor function on both hematopoietic and structural cells could also be relevant to the pathogenesis of AERD.

$PGE_2$ is generated primarily by COX-2 and a partner terminal synthetic enzyme, microsomal $PGE_2$ synthase 1 (mPGES-1). These 2 enzymes are coexpressed by epithelial cells, fibroblasts, and macrophages and are frequently upregulated in tandem during inflammatory responses.[61] There is substantial evidence that $PGE_2$ production and the functions of COX-2/mPGES-1 are impaired in the respiratory tissues in AERD. Although urinary levels of $PGE_2$ metabolites in AERD are similar to those in aspirin-tolerant controls, nasal polyps from patients with AERD contain markedly lower levels of $PGE_2$ than do sinonasal tissues from aspirin-tolerant individuals.[62] These levels are inversely related to the levels of cysLTs recovered from the same polyps. Peripheral blood leukocytes isolated from patients with AERD produce less $PGE_2$ than aspirin-tolerant controls,[63] and both nasal epithelial cells and cultured fibroblasts from nasal polyps of patients with AERD generate less $PGE_2$ in vitro than do cells from aspirin-tolerant asthmatic controls.[64,65] The expression of COX-2 mRNA is diminished in nasal polyps from patients with AERD compared with that in normal nasal mucosa and in polyps from aspirin-tolerant patients,[66] and the IL-1β-induced upregulation of COX-2 mRNA and protein expression in cultured fibroblasts from nasal polyps of patients with AERD is markedly blunted compared with their upregulation in cells from aspirin-tolerant controls.[65] Although there are no studies reporting the expression of mPGES-1 in AERD, the *PTGES* gene encoding this enzyme is hypermethylated (a mechanism for gene silencing) in nasal polyps from patients with AERD.[67] Collectively, these studies support defective function of the major system responsible for maintaining local $PGE_2$ in inflammation, potentially mediated by epigenetic mechanisms. A predicted outcome of the failure to appropriately upregulate COX-2 and mPGES-1 expression in the respiratory tissue is a dependency on COX-1 to provide the residual $PGE_2$ needed to maintain homeostasis of eosinophilic inflammation, mast cell activation, and 5-LO pathway activity. As noted later, this hypothetical dependency on COX-1 could contribute to a state of aspirin sensitivity.

## Alterations in $EP_2$ Receptor Expression and Function in AERD

Given the $EP_2$ receptor-dependent actions of $PGE_2$ noted earlier, it is noteworthy that the percentages of neutrophils, mast cells, eosinophils, and T cells expressing the $EP_2$ receptor are lower in nasal mucosa biopsies from patients with AERD compared with those in biopsies from aspirin-tolerant asthmatic controls.[68] Similar findings were recently reported for bronchial biopsies.[69] In addition, cultured fibroblasts from the nasal polyps of patients with AERD display decreased induction of the $EP_2$ receptor protein by IL-1β compared with fibroblasts from aspirin-tolerant patients.[65] Several SNPs in the promoter region of the $EP_2$ gene have been found to be associated with AERD, and the most significantly associated SNP, uS5, is located in the regulatory region of the $EP_2$ gene in a signal transducer and activator of transcription-binding consensus sequence and it confers reduced transcription activity.[70] However, this regulatory SNP was identified in only ~30% of patients with AERD versus ~20% of controls. The expression of $EP_2$ receptors (as well as that of COX-2) can become dysregulated by epigenetic mechanisms in cancer[71,72] and in pulmonary fibrosis.[73,74] It seems plausible that similar epigenetic mechanisms may promote deficiencies in these same targets in AERD, even in individuals who do not possess SNPs that dysregulate their expression.

### Other Arachidonic Acid Metabolites in AERD

Lipoxins (LXs) are unstable antiinflammatory derivatives of arachidonic acid, synthesized through transcellular mechanisms involving cooperation between 5-LO and platelet 12-LO[75] or 5-LO and epithelial cell-derived 15-LO.[76] In the presence of aspirin, COX-2 can function as a 15-LO and convert leukocyte-derived $LTA_4$ to 15-epi-$LXA_4$, also known as aspirin-triggered LX.[77] LXs inhibit cysLT production and eosinophilic infiltration of pulmonary tissue in rodent models of pulmonary inflammation,[78] and in vitro studies suggest that they are high-affinity antagonists of $CysLT_1R$.[79] Calcium ionophore stimulation of peripheral blood leukocytes from patients with AERD results in the release of less $LXA_4$ than does stimulation of leukocytes from the blood of aspirin-tolerant asthmatic control individuals.[80] Given the predicted antiinflammatory function of $LXA_4$, a deficient capacity to generate this mediator could contribute to the dysregulated inflammatory responses and cysLT-driven pathobiology of AERD, although this has not been validated in vivo.

### CROSS-TALK BETWEEN ARACHIDONIC ACID PATHWAYS IN THE PATHOBIOLOGY OF AERD AND GENESIS OF ASPIRIN-INDUCED REACTIONS

Although the events that initiate the development of AERD are unknown, the complex set of disturbances in the homeostasis of inflammation and lipid mediator production that characterize the basal state of the disease may hinge on a deficient synthesis of $PGE_2$ or on a diminished ability for it to signal through $EP_2$ receptors (**Fig. 3**). First, lowered levels of $PGE_2$ in the tissues combined with diminished expression of $EP_2$ receptors on the respiratory tissue granulocytes would allow for the dramatically elevated levels of cysLTs found in patients with AERD: it would permit enhanced $LTC_4$ synthesis by eosinophils and mast cells and would increase the neutrophil-derived $LTA_4$ available for conversion to $LTC_4$ by adherent platelets. Second, deficiencies in available $PGE_2$ and $EP_2$ receptor function would promote ongoing activation of mast cells and would remove a check on the chemotaxis of eosinophils. Third, $EP_2$ receptor signaling maintains TP receptors in a relative state of phosphorylation/desensitization via protein kinase A, and a recent study[59] revealed that $EP_2$ receptor signaling and mPGES-1-derived $PGE_2$ were essential to prevent exaggerated TP receptor-driven upregulation of endothelial cell ICAM-1 and consequent allergen-induced pulmonary eosinophilia and airway hyperreactivity. Last, deficient $EP_2$ receptor function on fibroblasts would impair the capacity of local $PGE_2$ to maintain a check on proliferation and collagen production. Thus, baseline impairment of local $PGE_2$ generation and $EP_2$ receptor signaling would likely promote persistent inflammation and ongoing tissue remodeling by several complementary mechanisms in AERD.

The defining respiratory reactions of AERD occur exclusively with drugs that inhibit COX isoforms nonselectively. At the low doses required to cause reactions in AERD, aspirin selectively inhibits the COX-1 isoenzyme[81] and it is inhibition of COX-1, but not of COX-2, which precipitates reactions.[82–85] All COX-1 inhibitors induce stereotypically similar respiratory reactions in patients with AERD, indicating that the ability of these structurally diverse drugs to inhibit COX-1 per se is via their pharmacologic actions. Although the basal state of AERD does not require exposure to COX inhibitors, the remarkable ability for low doses of aspirin (or any COX-1-active NSAID) to induce reactions implies that the aspirin sensitivity of AERD is caused by a tenuous dependency on COX-1 products to maintain homeostasis. Based on several lines of

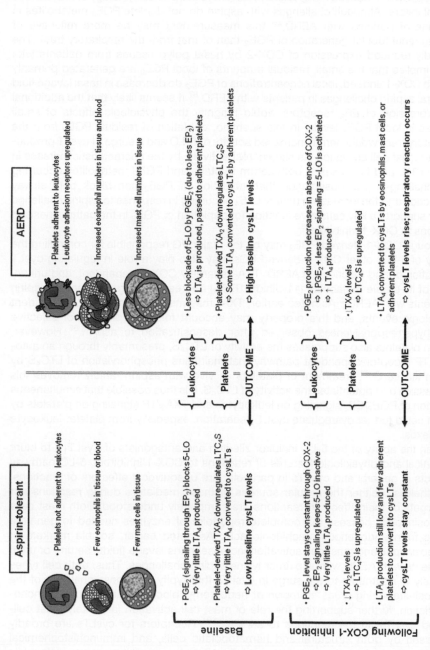

**Fig. 3.** Summary of the pathogenesis of AERD at baseline and after COX-1 inhibition. Normal mechanisms for the maintenance of homeostasis at baseline and after COX-1 inhibition in aspirin-tolerant control patients are presented on the left. The consequences of abnormalities that lead to both the underlying respiratory disease and the development of reactions on ingestion of COX-1 inhibitors in patients with AERD are presented on the right.

evidence, COX-1-derived $PGE_2$ is likely relevant to the pathophysiology of reactions to COX inhibitors. Although challenges with aspirin do not deplete $PGE_2$ metabolites in the urine of patients with AERD,[86] this measurement may be more reflective of ongoing renal tubular generation of $PGE_2$ than of that from the respiratory tract. The markedly reduced expression of COX-2 by nasal polyp tissues from patients with AERD implies that the small, residual amounts of local $PGE_2$ are generated primarily through COX-1. Indeed, local concentrations of $PGE_2$ do decrease in nasal lavage fluid after oral aspirin challenges in patients with AERD.[87] It seems likely that the additional low expression of $EP_2$ receptors would magnify the physiologic effects of small changes in local $PGE_2$ levels. In this scenario, depletion of residual $PGE_2$ from the respiratory tract would permit increased activity of 5-LO and a surge of cysLT production and mast cell activation (as shown, respectively, by the characteristic increase in urinary $LTE_4$ and increases in both serum tryptase and $PGD_2$ metabolites occurring after challenge). The observation that inhalation of $PGE_2$ can block both airway obstruction and the increase in urinary $LTE_4$ occurring in response to aspirin challenge further supports a key causative function for depletion of $PGE_2$ in the pathogenesis of reactions to COX-1 inhibitors.[57]

Although COX-1-derived $PGE_2$ may be the major PG responsible for controlling the activity of 5-LO, other COX-1-derived PGs may also play a role in regulating cysLT production during reactions in AERD. $TXA_2$ is largely COX-1-dependent, and urinary levels of its stable metabolite (11-dihidro $TXB_2$) decrease during reactions to aspirin in patients with AERD.[5] As noted earlier, $TXA_2$ may mediate certain $LTE_4$-dependent physiologic events, and this property may account for the rapid loss of selective $LTE_4$ hyperresponsiveness observed after desensitization to aspirin.[88] However, $TXA_2$ in platelets also suppresses the activity of $LTC_4S$, presumably through an autocrine, TP receptor-dependent pathway that maintains phosphorylation of $LTC_4S$ by protein kinase C.[89] Treatment of platelets ex vivo with aspirin rapidly removes this suppression and potentiates the activity of $LTC_4S$. It is thus possible that simultaneous depletion of $PGE_2/EP_2$ signaling on leukocytes and $TXA_2/TP$ signaling on platelets by aspirin could further dysregulate cysLT generation, especially from platelet-leukocyte complexes.

Given the ability of the 5-LO inhibitor zileuton and antagonists of $CysLT_1R$ to blunt the clinical and physiologic features of reactions to COX-1 inhibitors, 5-LO pathway products in general and cysLTs in particular are unequivocal effectors of reactions. Nevertheless, neither the cellular sources of these mediators during reactions nor the targets of their effects in reactions are completely understood. Both mast cells and eosinophils possess the complete repertoire of enzymes needed to generate cysLTs from endogenous arachidonic acid. As noted earlier, soluble markers of both eosinophil and mast cell activation increase in the lavage fluids, serum, or urine of patients with AERD with aspirin or lysine aspirin challenges. Thus, both cell types are likely to contribute to the surge in cysLTs that typify reactions. Inhalation of the mast cell-stabilizing drugs cromolyn or nedocromyl block aspirin-induced bronchoconstriction, further supporting the role of mast cell activation (and likely mast cell-derived cysLTs) in the reactions to aspirin.[90,91] Receptors for cysLTs are broadly expressed by both structural and hematopoietic cells, and immunohistochemical studies indicate that the expression of $CysLT_1R$ by respiratory tract eosinophils and mast cells is upregulated in AERD.[33] The administration of zileuton to subjects with AERD not only dramatically reduces the nasal symptoms of reactions to lysine aspirin challenge, but markedly reduces the concentrations of mast cell tryptase recovered from the nasal lavage fluid compared with the levels found in fluids from placebo-treated challenged controls.[24] It is thus likely that cysLTs induce a diverse array of physiologic effects during reactions beyond $CysLT_1R$-dependent broncho-constriction. The fact that $LTE_4$, the most abundant mediator detected during reactions, acts by receptors other than $CysLT_1R$ and $CysLT_2R$ makes this hypothesis a virtual certainty **Fig. 2**.

## SUMMARY

Physiologic and pharmacologic studies in humans strongly support the hypothesis that AERD involves fundamental disturbances in both the production of and end-organ responsiveness to eicosanoids that are regulators of homeostasis ($PGE_2$) and those that are effectors (cysLTs). The likelihood that these disturbances are acquired in adulthood implies potential epigenetic modifications of the relevant mediator systems as a result of only partially clarified environmental factors (eg, potentially viral or bacterial infections, inhaled pollutants). The rapid development of technology permitting analyses of the epigenetic landscape and the microbiome may permit finer detailing of the evasive causal agents and lesions. Meanwhile, the putative pathobiological mechanisms of AERD introduce substantial opportunities for targeted therapeutic intervention. The advent of anti-IL-5,[92] tyrosine kinase inhibitors,[93] and antiplatelet drugs[94] for other indications may permit novel therapeutic approaches to AERD by targeting some of the key cellular effectors (eosinophils, mast cells, platelets). Existing or new drugs that act by targeting of candidate mediators and receptors, such as $PGD_2/DP_2$[95] and $TXA_2/TP$,[96] should permit finer detail of their specific roles in disease pathogenesis, as well as providing additional potential efficacy of treatment. The anticipated identification of $LTE_4$-selective receptors and the development of $EP_2$ receptor-selective agonists have substantial therapeutic potential in AERD.

## REFERENCES

1. Szczeklik A, Nizankowska E, Duplaga M. Natural history of aspirin-induced asthma. AIANE Investigators. European Network on Aspirin-Induced Asthma. Eur Respir J 2000;16:432.
2. Adamjee J, Suh YJ, Park HS, et al. Expression of 5-lipoxygenase and cyclooxygenase pathway enzymes in nasal polyps of patients with aspirin-intolerant asthma. J Pathol 2006;209:392.
3. Cowburn AS, Sladek K, Soja J, et al. Overexpression of leukotriene C4 synthase in bronchial biopsies from patients with aspirin-intolerant asthma. J Clin Invest 1998;101:834.
4. Yamashita T, Tsuji H, Maeda N, et al. Etiology of nasal polyps associated with aspirin-sensitive asthma. Rhinol Suppl 1989;8:15.
5. Sladek K, Dworski R, Soja J, et al. Eicosanoids in bronchoalveolar lavage fluid of aspirin-intolerant patients with asthma after aspirin challenge. Am J Respir Crit Care Med 1994;149:940.
6. Hosemann W. Surgical treatment of nasal polyposis in patients with aspirin intolerance. Thorax 2000;55(Suppl 2):S87.
7. Kakoi H, Hiraide F. A histological study of formation and growth of nasal polyps. Acta Otolaryngol 1987;103:137.
8. Makowska JS, Grzegorczyk J, Bienkiewicz B, et al. Systemic responses after bronchial aspirin challenge in sensitive patients with asthma. J Allergy Clin Immunol 2008;121:348.

9. Laidlaw TM, Kidder MS, Bhattacharyya N, et al. Cysteinyl leukotriene overproduction in aspirin-exacerbated respiratory disease is driven by platelet-adherent leukocytes. Blood 2012;119:3790.
10. Hamilos DL, Leung DY, Wood R, et al. Evidence for distinct cytokine expression in allergic versus nonallergic chronic sinusitis. J Allergy Clin Immunol 1995;96:537.
11. Sousa AR, Lams BE, Pfister R, et al. Expression of interleukin-5 and granulocyte-macrophage colony-stimulating factor in aspirin-sensitive and non-aspirin-sensitive asthmatic airways. Am J Respir Crit Care Med 1997;156:1384.
12. Pearce N, Pekkanen J, Beasley R. How much asthma is really attributable to atopy? Thorax 1999;54:268.
13. Lee JY, Kim HM, Ye YM, et al. Role of staphylococcal superantigen-specific IgE antibodies in aspirin-intolerant asthma. Allergy Asthma Proc 2006;27:341.
14. Suh YJ, Yoon SH, Sampson AP, et al. Specific immunoglobulin E for staphylococcal enterotoxins in nasal polyps from patients with aspirin-intolerant asthma. Clin Exp Allergy 2004;34:1270.
15. Christie PE, Tagari P, Ford-Hutchinson AW, et al. Urinary leukotriene E4 concentrations increase after aspirin challenge in aspirin-sensitive asthmatic subjects. Am Rev Respir Dis 1991;143:1025.
16. Smith CM, Hawksworth RJ, Thien FC, et al. Urinary leukotriene E4 in bronchial asthma. Eur Respir J 1992;5:693.
17. Daffern PJ, Muilenburg D, Hugli TE, et al. Association of urinary leukotriene E4 excretion during aspirin challenges with severity of respiratory responses. J Allergy Clin Immunol 1999;104:559.
18. Dahlen SE, Hedqvist P, Hammarstrom S, et al. Leukotrienes are potent constrictors of human bronchi. Nature 1980;288:484.
19. Dahlen SE, Hansson G, Hedqvist P, et al. Allergen challenge of lung tissue from asthmatics elicits bronchial contraction that correlates with the release of leukotrienes C4, D4, and E4. Proc Natl Acad Sci U S A 1983;80:1712.
20. Dahlen SE, Bjork J, Hedqvist P, et al. Leukotrienes promote plasma leakage and leukocyte adhesion in postcapillary venules: in vivo effects with relevance to the acute inflammatory response. Proc Natl Acad Sci U S A 1981;78:3887.
21. Gauvreau GM, Parameswaran KN, Watson RM, et al. Inhaled leukotriene E(4), but not leukotriene D(4), increased airway inflammatory cells in subjects with atopic asthma. Am J Respir Crit Care Med 2001;164:1495.
22. Beller TC, Maekawa A, Friend DS, et al. Targeted gene disruption reveals the role of the cysteinyl leukotriene 2 receptor in increased vascular permeability and in bleomycin-induced pulmonary fibrosis in mice. J Biol Chem 2004;279:46129.
23. Henderson WR Jr, Tang LO, Chu SJ, et al. A role for cysteinyl leukotrienes in airway remodeling in a mouse asthma model. Am J Respir Crit Care Med 2002;165:108.
24. Fischer AR, Rosenberg MA, Lilly CM, et al. Direct evidence for a role of the mast cell in the nasal response to aspirin in aspirin-sensitive asthma. J Allergy Clin Immunol 1994;94:1046.
25. Dahlen SE, Malmstrom K, Nizankowska E, et al. Improvement of aspirin-intolerant asthma by montelukast, a leukotriene antagonist: a randomized, double-blind, placebo-controlled trial. Am J Respir Crit Care Med 2002;165:9.
26. Maclouf JA, Murphy RC. Transcellular metabolism of neutrophil-derived leukotriene A4 by human platelets. A potential cellular source of leukotriene C4. J Biol Chem 1988;263:174.

27. Maugeri N, Evangelista V, Celardo A, et al. Polymorphonuclear leukocyte-platelet interaction: role of P-selectin in thromboxane B2 and leukotriene C4 cooperative synthesis. Thromb Haemost 1994;72:450.

28. Sanak M, Pierzchalska M, Bazan-Socha S, et al. Enhanced expression of the leukotriene C(4) synthase due to overactive transcription of an allelic variant associated with aspirin-intolerant asthma. Am J Respir Cell Mol Biol 2000;23:290.

29. Van Sambeek R, Stevenson DD, Baldasaro M, et al. 5' flanking region polymorphism of the gene encoding leukotriene C4 synthase does not correlate with the aspirin-intolerant asthma phenotype in the United States. J Allergy Clin Immunol 2000;106:72.

30. Nasser SM, Pfister R, Christie PE, et al. Inflammatory cell populations in bronchial biopsies from aspirin-sensitive asthmatic subjects. Am J Respir Crit Care Med 1996;153:90.

31. Maekawa A, Kanaoka Y, Xing W, et al. Functional recognition of a distinct receptor preferential for leukotriene E4 in mice lacking the cysteinyl leukotriene 1 and 2 receptors. Proc Natl Acad Sci U S A 2008;105:16695.

32. Paruchuri S, Tashimo H, Feng C, et al. Leukotriene E4-induced pulmonary inflammation is mediated by the P2Y12 receptor. J Exp Med 2009;206:2543.

33. Sousa AR, Parikh A, Scadding G, et al. Leukotriene-receptor expression on nasal mucosal inflammatory cells in aspirin-sensitive rhinosinusitis. N Engl J Med 2002; 347:1493.

34. Kim SH, Oh JM, Kim YS, et al. Cysteinyl leukotriene receptor 1 promoter polymorphism is associated with aspirin-intolerant asthma in males. Clin Exp Allergy 2006;36:433.

35. Christie PE, Schmitz-Schumann M, Spur BW, et al. Airway responsiveness to leukotriene C4 (LTC4), leukotriene E4 (LTE4) and histamine in aspirin-sensitive asthmatic subjects. Eur Respir J 1993;6:1468.

36. Jiang Y, Borrelli LA, Kanaoka Y, et al. CysLT2 receptors interact with CysLT1 receptors and down-modulate cysteinyl leukotriene dependent mitogenic responses of mast cells. Blood 2007;110:3263.

37. Barrett NA, Fernandez JM, Maekawa A, et al. Cysteinyl leukotriene 2 receptor on dendritic cells negatively regulates ligand-dependent allergic pulmonary inflammation. J Immunol 2012;189:4556.

38. Park JS, Chang HS, Park CS, et al. Association analysis of cysteinyl-leukotriene receptor 2 (CYSLTR2) polymorphisms with aspirin intolerance in asthmatics. Pharmacogenet Genomics 2005;15:483.

39. DeWitt DL, el-Harith EA, Kraemer SA, et al. The aspirin and heme-binding sites of ovine and murine prostaglandin endoperoxide synthases. J Biol Chem 1990;265:5192.

40. Bureau MF, De Clerck F, Lefort J, et al. Thromboxane A2 accounts for bronchoconstriction but not for platelet sequestration and microvascular albumin exchanges induced by fMLP in the guinea pig lung. J Pharmacol Exp Ther 1992;260:832.

41. Ishizuka T, Kawakami M, Hidaka T, et al. Stimulation with thromboxane A2 (TXA2) receptor agonist enhances ICAM-1, VCAM-1 or ELAM-1 expression by human vascular endothelial cells. Clin Exp Immunol 1998;112:464.

42. Ueno A, Tanaka K, Katori M. Possible involvement of thromboxane in bronchoconstrictive and hypertensive effects of LTC4 and LTD4 in guinea pigs. Prostaglandins 1982;23:865.

43. Jacques CA, Spur BW, Johnson M, et al. The mechanism of LTE4-induced histamine hyperresponsiveness in guinea-pig tracheal and human bronchial smooth muscle, in vitro. Br J Pharmacol 1991;104:859.

44. Kim SH, Choi JH, Park HS, et al. Association of thromboxane A2 receptor gene polymorphism with the phenotype of acetyl salicylic acid-intolerant asthma. Clin Exp Allergy 2005;35:585.
45. Mita H, Endoh S, Kudoh M, et al. Possible involvement of mast-cell activation in aspirin provocation of aspirin-induced asthma. Allergy 2001;56:1061.
46. Bochenek G, Nagraba K, Nizankowska E, et al. A controlled study of 9alpha,11beta-PGF2 (a prostaglandin D2 metabolite) in plasma and urine of patients with bronchial asthma and healthy controls after aspirin challenge. J Allergy Clin Immunol 2003; 111:743.
47. Johnston SL, Freezer NJ, Ritter W, et al. Prostaglandin D2-induced bronchoconstriction is mediated only in part by the thromboxane prostanoid receptor. Eur Respir J 1995;8:411.
48. Larsson AK, Hagfjard A, Dahlen SE, et al. Prostaglandin D(2) induces contractions through activation of TP receptors in peripheral lung tissue from the guinea pig. Eur J Pharmacol 2011;669:136.
49. Hirai H, Tanaka K, Yoshie O, et al. Prostaglandin D2 selectively induces chemotaxis in T helper type 2 cells, eosinophils, and basophils via seven-transmembrane receptor CRTH2. J Exp Med 2001;193:255.
50. Sladek K, Szczeklik A. Cysteinyl leukotrienes overproduction and mast cell activation in aspirin-provoked bronchospasm in asthma. Eur Respir J 1993;6: 391.
51. Szczeklik A, Sladek K, Dworski R, et al. Bronchial aspirin challenge causes specific eicosanoid response in aspirin-sensitive asthmatics. Am J Respir Crit Care Med 1996;154:1608.
52. Sousa A, Pfister R, Christie PE, et al. Enhanced expression of cyclo-oxygenase isoenzyme 2 (COX-2) in asthmatic airways and its cellular distribution in aspirin-sensitive asthma. Thorax 1997;52:940.
53. Gauvreau GM, Watson RM, O'Byrne PM. Protective effects of inhaled PGE2 on allergen-induced airway responses and airway inflammation. Am J Respir Crit Care Med 1999;159:31.
54. Peachell PT, MacGlashan DW Jr, Lichtenstein LM, et al. Regulation of human basophil and lung mast cell function by cyclic adenosine monophosphate. J Immunol 1988;140:571.
55. Feng C, Beller EM, Bagga S, et al. Human mast cells express multiple EP receptors for prostaglandin E2 that differentially modulate activation responses. Blood 2006;107:3243.
56. Luo M, Jones SM, Flamand N, et al. Phosphorylation by protein kinase a inhibits nuclear import of 5-lipoxygenase. J Biol Chem 2005;280:40609.
57. Sestini P, Armetti L, Gambaro G, et al. Inhaled PGE2 prevents aspirin-induced bronchoconstriction and urinary LTE4 excretion in aspirin-sensitive asthma. Am J Respir Crit Care Med 1996;153:572.
58. Sturm EM, Schratl P, Schuligoi R, et al. Prostaglandin E2 inhibits eosinophil trafficking through E-prostanoid 2 receptors. J Immunol 2008;181:7273.
59. Liu T, Laidlaw TM, Feng C, et al. Prostaglandin E2 deficiency uncovers a dominant role for thromboxane A2 in house dust mite-induced allergic pulmonary inflammation. Proc Natl Acad Sci U S A 2012;109:12692.
60. Huang SK, Wettlaufer SH, Hogaboam CM, et al. Variable prostaglandin E2 resistance in fibroblasts from patients with usual interstitial pneumonia. Am J Respir Crit Care Med 2008;177:66.
61. Uematsu S, Matsumoto M, Takeda K, et al. Lipopolysaccharide-dependent prostaglandin E(2) production is regulated by the glutathione-dependent prostaglandin

E(2) synthase gene induced by the Toll-like receptor 4/MyD88/NF-IL6 pathway. J Immunol 2002;168:5811.

62. Yoshimura T, Yoshikawa M, Otori N, et al. Correlation between the prostaglandin D(2)/E(2) ratio in nasal polyps and the recalcitrant pathophysiology of chronic rhinosinusitis associated with bronchial asthma. Allergol Int 2008;57:429.

63. Schafer D, Schmid M, Gode UC, et al. Dynamics of eicosanoids in peripheral blood cells during bronchial provocation in aspirin-intolerant asthmatics. Eur Respir J 1999;13:638.

64. Kowalski ML, Pawliczak R, Wozniak J, et al. Differential metabolism of arachidonic acid in nasal polyp epithelial cells cultured from aspirin-sensitive and aspirin-tolerant patients. Am J Respir Crit Care Med 2000;161:391.

65. Roca-Ferrer J, Garcia-Garcia FJ, Pereda J, et al. Reduced expression of COXs and production of prostaglandin E(2) in patients with nasal polyps with or without aspirin-intolerant asthma. J Allergy Clin Immunol 2011;128:66.

66. Picado C, Fernandez-Morata JC, Juan M, et al. Cyclooxygenase-2 mRNA is downexpressed in nasal polyps from aspirin-sensitive asthmatics. Am J Respir Crit Care Med 1999;160:291.

67. Cheong HS, Park SM, Kim MO, et al. Genome-wide methylation profile of nasal polyps: relation to aspirin hypersensitivity in asthmatics. Allergy 2011;66:637.

68. Ying S, Meng Q, Scadding G, et al. Aspirin-sensitive rhinosinusitis is associated with reduced E-prostanoid 2 receptor expression on nasal mucosal inflammatory cells. J Allergy Clin Immunol 2006;117:312.

69. Corrigan CJ, Napoli RL, Meng Q, et al. Reduced expression of the prostaglandin E2 receptor E-prostanoid 2 on bronchial mucosal leukocytes in patients with aspirin-sensitive asthma. J Allergy Clin Immunol 2012;129:1636.

70. Jinnai N, Sakagami T, Sekigawa T, et al. Polymorphisms in the prostaglandin E2 receptor subtype 2 gene confer susceptibility to aspirin-intolerant asthma: a candidate gene approach. Hum Mol Genet 2004;13:3203.

71. Gray SG, Al-Sarraf N, Baird AM, et al. Regulation of EP receptors in non-small cell lung cancer by epigenetic modifications. Eur J Cancer 2009;45:3087.

72. de Maat MF, van de Velde CJ, Umetani N, et al. Epigenetic silencing of cyclooxygenase-2 affects clinical outcome in gastric cancer. J Clin Oncol 2007; 25:4887.

73. Huang SK, Fisher AS, Scruggs AM, et al. Hypermethylation of PTGER2 confers prostaglandin E2 resistance in fibrotic fibroblasts from humans and mice. Am J Pathol 2010;177:2245.

74. Coward WR, Watts K, Feghali-Bostwick CA, et al. Defective histone acetylation is responsible for the diminished expression of cyclooxygenase 2 in idiopathic pulmonary fibrosis. Mol Cell Biol 2009;29:4325.

75. Serhan CN, Sheppard KA. Lipoxin formation during human neutrophil-platelet interactions. Evidence for the transformation of leukotriene A4 by platelet 12-lipoxygenase in vitro. J Clin Invest 1990;85:772.

76. Edenius C, Kumlin M, Bjork T, et al. Lipoxin formation in human nasal polyps and bronchial tissue. FEBS Lett 1990;272:25.

77. Takano T, Fiore S, Maddox JF, et al. Aspirin-triggered 15-epi-lipoxin A4 (LXA4) and LXA4 stable analogues are potent inhibitors of acute inflammation: evidence for anti-inflammatory receptors. J Exp Med 1997;185:1693.

78. Levy BD, De Sanctis GT, Devchand PR, et al. Multi-pronged inhibition of airway hyper-responsiveness and inflammation by lipoxin A(4). Nat Med 2002;8:1018.

79. Gronert K, Martinsson-Niskanen T, Ravasi S, et al. Selectivity of recombinant human leukotriene D(4), leukotriene B(4), and lipoxin A(4) receptors with

aspirin-triggered 15-epi-LXA(4) and regulation of vascular and inflammatory responses. Am J Pathol 2001;158:3.

80. Sanak M, Levy BD, Clish CB, et al. Aspirin-tolerant asthmatics generate more lipoxins than aspirin-intolerant asthmatics. Eur Respir J 2000;16:44.

81. Meade EA, Smith WL, DeWitt DL. Differential inhibition of prostaglandin endoperoxide synthase (cyclooxygenase) isozymes by aspirin and other non-steroidal anti-inflammatory drugs. J Biol Chem 1993;268:6610.

82. Yoshida S, Ishizaki Y, Onuma K, et al. Selective cyclo-oxygenase 2 inhibitor in patients with aspirin-induced asthma. J Allergy Clin Immunol 2000;106:1201.

83. Szczeklik A, Nizankowska E, Bochenek G, et al. Safety of a specific COX-2 inhibitor in aspirin-induced asthma. Clin Exp Allergy 2001;31:219.

84. Dahlen B, Szczeklik A, Murray JJ. Celecoxib in patients with asthma and aspirin intolerance. The Celecoxib in Aspirin-Intolerant Asthma Study Group. N Engl J Med 2001;344:142.

85. Stevenson DD, Simon RA. Lack of cross-reactivity between rofecoxib and aspirin in aspirin-sensitive patients with asthma. J Allergy Clin Immunol 2001;108:47.

86. Mastalerz L, Sanak M, Gawlewicz-Mroczka A, et al. Prostaglandin E2 systemic production in patients with asthma with and without aspirin hypersensitivity. Thorax 2008;63:27.

87. Ferreri NR, Howland WC, Stevenson DD, et al. Release of leukotrienes, prostaglandins, and histamine into nasal secretions of aspirin-sensitive asthmatics during reaction to aspirin. Am Rev Respir Dis 1988;137:847.

88. Arm JP, O'Hickey SP, Spur BW, et al. Airway responsiveness to histamine and leukotriene E4 in subjects with aspirin-induced asthma. Am Rev Respir Dis 1989;140:148.

89. Tornhamre S, Ehnhage A, Kolbeck KG, et al. Uncoupled regulation of leukotriene C4 synthase in platelets from aspirin-intolerant asthmatics and healthy volunteers after aspirin treatment. Clin Exp Allergy 2002;32:1566.

90. Yoshida S, Amayasu H, Sakamoto H, et al. Cromolyn sodium prevents bronchoconstriction and urinary LTE4 excretion in aspirin-induced asthma. Ann Allergy Asthma Immunol 1998;80:171.

91. Robuschi M, Gambaro G, Sestini P, et al. Attenuation of aspirin-induced bronchoconstriction by sodium cromoglycate and nedocromil sodium. Am J Respir Crit Care Med 1997;155:1461.

92. O'Byrne PM. The demise of anti IL-5 for asthma, or not. Am J Respir Crit Care Med 2007;176:1059.

93. Pardanani A, Elliott M, Reeder T, et al. Imatinib for systemic mast-cell disease. Lancet 2003;362:535.

94. Wiviott SD, Braunwald E, McCabe CH, et al. Prasugrel versus clopidogrel in patients with acute coronary syndromes. N Engl J Med 2007;357:2001.

95. Uller L, Mathiesen JM, Alenmyr L, et al. Antagonism of the prostaglandin D2 receptor CRTH2 attenuates asthma pathology in mouse eosinophilic airway inflammation. Respir Res 2007;8:16.

96. Zuccollo A, Shi C, Mastroianni R, et al. The thromboxane A2 receptor antagonist S18886 prevents enhanced atherogenesis caused by diabetes mellitus. Circulation 2005;112:3001.

# Aspirin Desensitization in Aspirin-Exacerbated Respiratory Disease

Andrew A. White, MD*, Donald D. Stevenson, MD

## KEYWORDS

- Aspirin • Aspirin desensitization • COX-1 inhibitors
- Leukotriene-modifying drugs (LTMDs) • Oral aspirin challenges (OAC)

## KEY POINTS

- All patients with aspirin-exacerbated respiratory disease can be desensitized to aspirin.
- All nonsteroidal anti-inflammatory drugs that are competitive inhibitors of cyclooxygenase-1 have been shown to cross-desensitize with aspirin.
- Therapeutic benefits to patients with aspirin-exacerbated respiratory disease who continue daily aspirin include the following:
  - A decrease in nasal polyp formation, nasal congestion, sinus infections, sinus surgery, and need for systemic corticosteroids.
  - An increase in asthma control and sense of smell.

## HISTORY OF ASPIRIN DESENSITIZATION

In 1922, Fernand Widal, Pierre Abrami, and Jaques Lemoyez[1] published an article that explored all the clinical issues surrounding aspirin-exacerbated respiratory disease (AERD). This article was translated into English by Amy D. Klion, MD in 1993.[2] Professor Fernand Widal was appointed Chairman of Clinical Medicine at l'Hopital Cochin in Paris in 1917 and was already an expert on bacterial infections, particularly streptococcus and salmonella. Professor Widal and his coauthors were the first to describe the clinical presentation of AERD and the reaction to aspirin, which was at the time inappropriately diagnosed as "anaphylaxis." All of their observations evolved out of 1 case report.

This case report concerned a 37-year-old woman, who, at age 26 (in 1910), developed nasal polyps, intermittent urticarial swellings, and, later, asthma. Her major symptoms

Disclosures: None.
Division of Allergy and Immunology, The Scripps Research Institute, Scripps Clinic, 3811 Valley Centre Drive, San Diego, CA 92130, USA
* Corresponding author.
E-mail address: White.Andrew@scrippshealth.org

Immunol Allergy Clin N Am 33 (2013) 211–222
http://dx.doi.org/10.1016/j.iac.2012.10.013
0889-8561/13/$ – see front matter © 2013 Elsevier Inc. All rights reserved.

immunology.theclinics.com

were nasal obstruction with continuous postnasal drainage. Per the report, "A specialist found and ablated mucous polyps in the nasal pharynx in 1913 and for several months the patient had no further sneezing or runny nose." As the years went by, increasing asthma attacks, lasting weeks at a time, were particularly likely to occur in the winter "when there was no pollen in the air." In 1921, the patient was admitted to the hospital and underwent extensive investigations. The state of her asthma activity was not apparent from the article but in 1922 there were no controller medications for asthma. She underwent an oral challenge with 10 centigrains (0.1 grain) of aspirin. One grain is equivalent to 64.798 mg. Therefore, the initial dose of aspirin was 6.5 mg, given at 12:15 PM. By 1:30 PM, generalized urticaria occurred. At 2 PM, an asthma attack started and continued until "the evening." At 3:40 PM, the urticaria disappeared as the patient developed "serial sneezing and nasal hydrorrhea," which continued into the night. The next day, "the patient was exhausted" but all of her respiratory and cutaneous symptoms "vanished." An identical reaction occurred to antipyrine, the only other nonsteroidal anti-inflammatory drug (NSAID) available at the time. Oral challenges, with drugs that did not inhibit cyclooxygenase, namely chlorohydrate of quinine, urotropine, or pyramidon, "did not induce this previously described reaction."

The authors then reasoned that these "idiosyncratic episodes and their striking similarity to drug induced anaphylaxis" might be made to disappear by the same procedure of "desensitization" used in a prior case of "antipyrine anaphylaxis." They started daily ingestion of 1 cg (6.5 mg) of aspirin, and every 4 days increased by 1 cg up to 5 cg (32.5 mg) of aspirin, which produced no symptoms. Two months later, after slowly increasing aspirin doses, the patient could ingest 60 cg (390 mg) of aspirin each day without any adverse effect. She was then challenged with antipyrine, "a substance to which the patient had been equally intolerant" during a prior oral challenge. The authors then reported that "...despite their considerable difference in chemical nature, we were very surprised to find that desensitization to aspirin led to concomitant desensitization to antipyrine, a phenomenon not seen in anaphylaxis." Unfortunately, after completing these experiments, the authors did not prescribe daily aspirin for the patient.

These remarkable descriptions and experimental oral challenges established the following:

1. AERD was a disease of nasal polyposis and asthma with onset at age 26 years old.
2. Removal of polyps improved the disease temporarily.
3. During the winter, the patient experienced severe and prolonged asthma attacks when there was no pollen in the air (viral-induced asthma exacerbations in an AERD patient).
4. During asthma remission, a low dose (6.5 mg) of aspirin, in a completely untreated and unprotected asthmatic patient, produced transient hives, prolonged and severe bronchospasm, and profound nasal discharge. (The patient survived because Professor Widal had the good sense to start the oral challenge with a very low dose of aspirin.)
5. By the next day the patient was "exhausted" (a classic finding after an aspirin-induced respiratory reaction).
6. With desensitization, 390 mg aspirin daily could be ingested without adverse effects.
7. Although, at the time, the mechanism of cyclooxygenase-1 (COX-1) inhibition was not recognized, medical professionals now know that antipyrine is a COX-1 inhibitor. Cross-desensitization to antipyrine, a structurally completely different drug, was demonstrated, providing the first example of NSAID cross-desensitization.

It is truly amazing that through the willingness of the patient to participate, and the scientific insight of Professor Widal, many of the fundamental aspects of AERD were identified decades before any subsequent investigations took place. Unfortunately for the patient, Professor Widal did not know that continuing daily aspirin at a dose of 390 mg or more would have been a therapeutic blessing for his AERD patient who, in the 1920s, had no other therapeutic options.

It was not until the 1970s that interest and research into AERD gained momentum. Several studies better characterized the reaction to aspirin and patient characteristics. In 1976, Zeiss and Lockey[3] reported a 72-hour refractory period to aspirin after a positive oral challenge with indomethacin. In 1977, Bianco and colleagues[4] challenged an AERD patient with inhaled aspirin lysine, which induced an asthmatic response. For the next 72 hours, inhalation of the same provoking doses of acetylsalicylic acid (ASA)-lysine did not induce any bronchospasm. In 1982, the refractory period, following aspirin desensitization, was studied in detail.[5] It was observed that in all 30 AERD patients, a 48-hour refractory period occurred following an aspirin-induced respiratory reaction. Furthermore, between 48 hours and 96 hours, the refractory period waned and all patients became vulnerable to a second aspirin challenge, which again induced a respiratory reaction.

In 1980, Stevenson and colleagues[6] made the serendipitous discovery that, after an oral aspirin challenge with 325 mg aspirin had induced a significant respiratory reaction, not only did a refractory period to aspirin ensue but also patients' nasal congestion disappeared and this state of desensitization could be maintained with 325 mg daily aspirin. Over the next year, treatment with daily aspirin in 2 patients with AERD induced significant remissions in their underlying respiratory disease and at the same time allowed discontinuation of prednisone in 1 patient and a 50% reduction in methylprednisolone in the second patient. This observation propelled AERD desensitization research into its next phase.

## SAFETY AND EFFICACY OF ASPIRIN DESENSITIZATION FOLLOWED BY DAILY TREATMENT WITH ASPIRIN

A 1983 study of 19 patients was the first to show that AERD could exist as only a sinonasal disease, without any associated asthma.[7] The absence of asthma was based on history, normal lung function values, and no decline in forced expiratory volume ($FEV_1$) values during methacholine inhalation challenges. Oral aspirin challenges induced only upper airway reactions (sneezing, rhinorrhea, nasal congestion, and ocular injection) with no asthma symptoms or changes in pulmonary function values. After the aspirin-induced reactions, nasal aspirin desensitization was induced in all 19 patients. Seventeen patients were treated with daily aspirin 650 mg twice a day for a year or more and 13 of 17 (77%) patients gained significant improvement in their nasal symptoms.

In 1984, the first (and only) randomized double-blind placebo-controlled crossover trial in AERD patients was published.[8] In this study, 25 patients underwent aspirin desensitization and during the 3-month aspirin treatment arm reported significant improvement in their nasal symptoms. Half of the patients experienced improvement in asthma symptoms during active treatment. Retrospectively, many of the patients in this 1981 to 1983 study correctly volunteered that they knew when they were in their 3 months of placebo versus aspirin treatment months. Even in this enormously difficult study, where re-desensitization was required in the middle of the study and every attempt was made to blind the placebo arm with identical placebo tablets, many of the study participants could not be blinded, because the immediate and sustained effect of aspirin on nasal decongestion is usually obvious.

The only other blinded controlled study was conducted in Germany and published in 2008.[9] This group of ear, nose, and throat surgeons carefully inspected the nasal cavities before and after aspirin desensitization. AERD patients were randomly assigned to daily aspirin treatment with 100 mg once a day or 300 mg once a day. Patients in the low-treatment arm, using 100 mg aspirin daily, experienced no benefit over the study year, but patients taking 300 mg of aspirin once a day did not reform nasal polyps and recorded effective control over nasal and sinus symptoms. This study circumvented the problem of a placebo arm and showed that, while aspirin desensitization could be maintained with 100 mg aspirin daily, such a low dose of aspirin was ineffective in controlling mucosal inflammation.

## LONG-TERM CONFIRMATORY STUDIES DEMONSTRATING EFFICACY OF ASPIRIN DESENSITIZATION

As chronic treatment with aspirin in AERD was now becoming recognized as a potential new and innovative treatment of AERD in the 1980s, larger confirmatory studies on long-term efficacy and side effects were necessary. Three long-term, open prospective studies were performed at Scripps Clinic between 1980 and 2000.

The first was published in 1990, where 107 known AERD patients were recruited.[10] There were 3 groups of patients: 42 avoided aspirin and served as controls; 35 were desensitized with aspirin and treated with aspirin 650 mg twice a day for a mean of 3.75 years (range, 1–8 years); 30 were treated with ASA 650 mg twice a day for 2 years and then discontinued aspirin. Compared with the control group, both ASA-treated groups were significantly improved (across multiple outcomes of sense of smell, asthma, sinus surgery requirements, and corticosteroid requirements).

The second study, published in 1996, enrolled 65 patients with known AERD.[11] This study was designed to see if, over time, the therapeutic effects of aspirin desensitization declined during long-term treatment. Using pre-desensitization years as the baseline, patients were divided into treatment groups for 1 to 3 years (29 patients) and 3 to 6 years (36 patients). All outcomes described in the 1990 article mentioned earlier were again recorded for both groups without any deterioration in the 3- to 6-year subgroup. Need for additional sinus or polyp surgery continued to be delayed past the 6-year study period, suggesting that long-term prevention of polyp formation continued.

The third study was published in 2003 and consisted of 172 consecutive patients with documented AERD.[12] After aspirin desensitization, all patients were treated with aspirin 650 mg twice a day and followed with monthly telephone surveys for 6 months and then biannually for up to 6 years. At 6 months, an improvement in numbers of sinus infections, sense of smell, nasal symptoms, and asthma symptom scores was seen. By 1 year, a decrease in rates of admission for asthma, emergency room visits for asthma, and sinus surgeries was noted in the aspirin-treated patients when compared with their own historical data collected in the year before desensitization. Importantly, at both 6 and 12 months, a significant decrease in the use of systemic and topical corticosteroids was recorded (10.8 mg once a day to 8.1 mg once a day and at 1 year 3.6 mg once a day). In this study, an intention-to-treat analysis provided an accurate assessment of the benefits of aspirin therapy. Of the 172 patients, 115 (67%) patients responded positively to aspirin treatment and 24 (14%) patients discontinued aspirin because of known aspirin side effects (mostly abdominal pain or bleeding). Five patients, who responded to aspirin, ultimately discontinued aspirin because of elective surgery or pregnancy. In another 17 patients (11%), their physicians discontinued aspirin for various reasons that were not intrinsically related to aspirin itself (entering another medical study, increase in liver function tests, asthmatic flare during a viral lower respiratory tract infection, etc). Of the remaining 126 patients, who completed a year of aspirin treatment without side effects or inappropriately discontinued aspirin treatment, 110 (87%)

patients experienced clinical improvement as outlined previously. Thus, it can be concluded from this study that most of the patients who undergo aspirin desensitization and continue daily aspirin therapy will gain benefit. Of the 16 patients who failed aspirin desensitization, 14 had concomitant allergic rhinitis with a high prevalence of dust mite and home pet allergy exposure.

During the informed consent discussion of the risks and benefits of aspirin desensitization, patients can be counseled that between 67% and 87% will both tolerate and gain benefit from daily aspirin therapy. Unfortunately, 13% of all patients treated daily with aspirin will obtain benefit to their respiratory tract, but will be unable to continue aspirin therapy because of side effects. These pivotal studies brought the use of aspirin therapy in AERD into the forefront of treatment of AERD patients with recalcitrant sinus/polyp disease. They have given clinicians a framework for discussion with patients regarding reasonable expectations of long-term, high-dose aspirin therapy.

In the most recent dose ranging study, 137 known AERD patients were randomized to take aspirin 325 mg twice a day or 650 mg twice a day after completing aspirin desensitization.[13] Prior studies suggested that aspirin at doses lower than 325 mg per day were unlikely to provide benefit to the patient, yet it was unclear what the optimal aspirin dose to treat AERD might be. In this Scripps Clinic study,[13] approximately 50% of patients randomized to the lower dose arm required an increase to the higher dose arm at 1 month because of incomplete nasal patency. Conversely, 50% of the subjects in the high-dose treatment arm were able to decrease their dose to 325 mg twice daily at 1 month without any change in their already documented clinical improvement. Surprisingly, the prevalence of known side effects, particularly gastritis and bleeding, was the same in both study groups. This study highlighted 2 important findings, namely, that the dose of aspirin necessary to treat AERD varies from patient to patient and that the side effects are the same in both dose ranges. It remains uncertain why higher doses of aspirin are necessary to elicit a clinical response in AERD. Aspirin's ability to inhibit COX-1 or COX-2 enzymes (81 mg once a day) seems to be too low to have significant therapeutic effects in patients with AERD.[9] It is likely that aspirin acts in decreasing inflammation in AERD through an as yet unknown off target mechanism.

## EARLY EFFECTS OF ASPIRIN DESENSITIZATION AND DAILY TREATMENT WITH ASPIRIN

In a 1986 study, Kowalski and colleagues[14] conducted oral aspirin challenges in 16 patients, desensitized them to aspirin, and then treated them with aspirin 600 mg once a day for 4 weeks. Gastritis developed in 4 patients, who dropped out. At the end of the treatment month, in the remaining 12 patients, marked reduction in nasal and asthma symptom scores, reduction in beta-agonist use, and bronchial responsiveness to inhaled histamine were observed.

In the authors' 2003 study, similar results were recorded at 1-month post aspirin desensitization treatment with aspirin 650 mg twice a day.[15] At 4 weeks, compared with baseline data, nasal and asthma symptom scores improved significantly. For the 15 patients taking prednisone at entry, the mean dose could be decreased from 10.7 mg once a day at baseline to 5.9 mg by the end of the first month. It is clear that the long-term benefits of aspirin therapy are present at 1 month and likely begin to emerge in the first few days to weeks of aspirin therapy.

## THE USE OF MEDICATIONS TO ENHANCE SAFETY OF ASPIRIN CHALLENGE/DESENSITIZATION AND TREATMENT

By 2006, aspirin desensitization was a standard treatment throughout the world and data on potential mechanisms (see article in this issue on Mechanisms of Aspirin

Desensitization), refinement of methods, challenge locations, and protocols were evolving. Based on the authors' early protocols,[16] most patients were admitted to the hospital (General Clinical Research Center at Scripps Clinic) while taking their usual asthma controller medications. Antihistamines were withheld because concomitant antihistamine treatment during oral aspirin challenges (OAC) could block cutaneous and nasal reactions, leading to false-negative challenges (**Table 1**).[17] On the first day, patients underwent oral placebo challenges to verify stable pulmonary function. On day 2, patients began to receive initial aspirin doses of 30 mg, 45 mg, or 60 mg, followed by advancing doses of 60 mg or 100 mg, 150 mg, 325 mg, and 650 mg with all dosing 3 hours apart. An intravenous line was routinely started before the desensitization. Serial spirometry was performed during OAC. A fairly typical threshold dose of approximately 60 mg aspirin induced reactions in most patients. After the patient reacted, appropriate treatment was initiated, and after recovery, the threshold aspirin dose was repeated. Although subsequent reactions could occur at higher doses of aspirin, these usually were less intense and easy to treat. The average patient would require 4 to 5 days of active aspirin dosing during a positive OAC.

After the appearance of leukotriene-modifying drugs (LTMDs) between 1998 and 1999, interest in using these drugs for broncho-protection was obvious. During OAC, the terminal leukotriene ($LTE_4$) appears in the urine approximately 2 to 6 hours after the respiratory reaction.[18,19] The more severe the aspirin-induced bronchospasm, the greater the concentration of urinary $LTE_4$.[19] This underscored the relative importance of initiating cysteinyl leukotriene receptor blockade during OAC.

Three studies conducted at the Scripps Clinic between 2002 and 2006 shed light on this subject. The first determined whether concomitant treatment with LTMDs was associated with a reduction in ASA-induced lower respiratory tract reactions, when compared with a control group who were not taking LTMDs.[20] In the LTMD-treated group, 96 patients were taking leukotriene receptor antagonists and 12 were taking zileuton. In the control group, without treatment, there were 163 patients. Results showed a strongly significant decrease in lower respiratory tract reactions and an increase in nasal reactors alone in the leukotriene receptor antagonists–protected patients. Similar results of broncho-protection were recorded for the12 zileuton-protected patients. Thus, some of the pure nasal reactors would have been classic

| Table 1 | | |
| --- | --- | --- |
| Sample oral aspirin challenge/desensitization protocol for AERD | | |
| Time | Day 1[a] | Day 2 |
| 8 AM | 20–40 mg[b] | 100–160 mg |
| 11 AM | 40–60 mg | 160–325 mg |
| 2 PM | 60–100 mg | 325 mg[c] |

(1) Measure $FEV_1$ every hour and wait 3 h between doses. (2) $FEV_1$ should be at least 1.5 L and >60% of predicted. (3) Reactions can be (a) naso-ocular alone; (b) naso-ocular and a 15% or greater decline in $FEV_1$ (Classic reaction); (c) lower respiratory reaction only ($FEV_1$ declines by >20%); (d) laryngospasm with or without a, b, or c (flat or notched inspiratory curve); (e) systemic reaction: hives, flush, gastric pain, hypotension. (4) Aspirin desensitization: (a) After a reaction has been treated and the reaction has subsided, that provoking dose should be repeated; (b) if no reaction, continue to escalate the doses as listed above.

  [a] A placebo challenge can be conducted the day before actual challenge begins if baseline unstable airways are suspected.

  [b] Aspirin doses can be prepared in advance by a compounding pharmacy. A simple alternative would to use a pill cutter; 81 mg ASA tablet can be cut into one-half or one-fourth.

  [c] For subjects who do not react to any dose including the 325 mg dose, it is not necessary to challenge with 650 mg of aspirin because this will also be negative.

upper and lower airway reactors, without the LTMD blockade of their bronchial cysteinyl leukotriene 1 receptors.

In the second study, using a large cohort of 678 AERD patients (1981–2004), the authors were able to also examine the effects of different controller medications on the presence and severity of lower respiratory reactions during oral aspirin challenges.[21] Thus, in addition to LTMDs, inhaled and systemic corticosteroids and long-acting beta-agonists were evaluated as to their effects on lower respiratory reactions. Somewhat surprisingly, although corticosteroids and long-acting bronchodilators stabilized baseline bronchoreactivity, they did not significantly blunt aspirin-induced bronchospasm, whereas LTMDs did. Importantly, the number of negative challenges in those taking LTMDs was reasonably small. However, these studies consistently demonstrated a worrisome rate of negative challenge of approximately 11% to 15%, suggesting that some patients enjoyed complete blockade of the respiratory tract, with false-negative reactions, while proceeding to silent desensitization.[22]

The third study, published in 2006, was designed to look at whether LTMDs could reduce not only the incidence of lower respiratory tract asthmatic reactions[20,21] but also the severity of reactions in the patients who did experience aspirin-induced asthma attacks despite pretreatment with LTMDs.[23] In this study of 676 patients with AERD, the addition of an LTMD (almost always montelukast) significantly reduced the severity (as measured by $FEV_1$ values) of aspirin-induced bronchospasm in those patients experiencing asthmatic reactions, compared with non-LTMD-treated control AERD patients. On the other hand, systemic corticosteroids, inhaled corticosteroids, and beta-agonists did not influence the severity of aspirin-induced bronchospasm. These studies led to the recommendation of montelukast pretreatment for several days before and during aspirin desensitization in all patients, unless a compelling contraindication exists.

## CURRENT PRACTICES IN THE PERFORMANCE OF ASPIRIN DESENSITIZATION AND ASPIRIN TREATMENT

Until the early 2000s, aspirin desensitization remained a highly specialized procedure relegated to allergy centers in only a few locations around the world. This relegation was because of concerns over safety and logistics. Over the past decade, many studies and guidelines have now made it much easier for the general allergist to perform desensitization in the outpatient clinic. In terms of safety, the authors know that previous historical reactions to aspirin or NSAIDs do not predict the severity of asthmatic reactions during oral aspirin challenge/desensitization,[24] as explained by several factors. Historical reactions were to full therapeutic doses of NSAIDS or aspirin; LTMD treatment was unusual and stable asthma may not have been present. During OACs, a subthreshold dose of aspirin was given with protective effects of LTMD and baseline asthma control was assured.[20,21] Because the respiratory reaction is dose dependent and LTMDs block asthma responses in half the patients and blunt them in the other half of the patients, an OAC is completely different from a casual ingestion of full-dose aspirin. This study and the experience have led to the successful migration of aspirin challenge/desensitization from an inpatient setting to the outpatient setting. In fact, the use of an inpatient or intensive care unit level of care adds unneeded burdens of complexity and expense to conduction of aspirin challenge/desensitization. For the past decade, the authors have consistently found that performing aspirin desensitization in the outpatient setting has been safe, successful, and cost effective. In the outpatient setting, it is important to place the patient in a central location, easily visible to nursing staff, and to have experienced nurses attending and frequently monitoring the patient. In the minds of some physicians, the issue of safety represents a barrier to recommending or performing desensitization, but the authors think that they have overcome this issue. Alternatively, there are now enough aspirin desensitization centers in the United States to make local or regional referrals an option for those allergy specialists who would rarely perform this procedure.

It is recognized that aspirin desensitization is not risk free or without safety concerns. All patients must be screened for stable bronchial airways before desensitization. Obviously, the worst case situation would be severe asthma leading to respiratory failure. Fortunately, since the routine use of LTMDs during desensitization, acute respiratory failure has not occurred during a controlled aspirin challenge/desensitization. Indeed, after the introduction of montelukast in 1999, no patients were moved to an intensive care unit or nor was intubation considered in any instance. Nonetheless, judicious use of inhaled corticosteroids, long-acting beta-agonists, and systemic corticosteroids should be considered in all patients. For most patients, a baseline $FEV_1$ of greater than 1.5 L is recommended before beginning aspirin desensitization.

After an aspirin challenge is positive (see article on AERD: Clinical Disease and Diagnosis) and symptoms have resolved, the provoking dose can be repeated and desensitization can proceed. The authors learned from their 2009 study that if the challenges are negative after the 325 mg aspirin dose, further challenges with 650 mg aspirin will not recruit any more aspirin-positive patients.[25] This information is useful from a practical standpoint because protocols can stop at 325 mg and save 3 hours of challenge time.

After the first reaction to aspirin, while repeating the offending dose, the patient (and sometimes the physician) may be hesitant to proceed but further dosing invariably leads to a muted reaction or more commonly is not associated with any further symptoms or reactions. The ability to attain acute desensitization is a nearly universal phenomenon and should be expected by the patient and treating physician. The authors reported 1 case of a patient who continued to react to 650 mg aspirin with reproducible bronchospasm, thus making ongoing treatment with aspirin an untenable proposition.[26]

The only other situation that limits a successful acute desensitization is urticaria. Previous studies have outlined the difficulty in trying to desensitize patients to aspirin with underlying chronic urticaria.[27] Rare patients have coexistent AERD and chronic urticaria. Although desensitization can safely be attempted in this group, it should be anticipated that protracted and difficult to control urticaria may make long-term aspirin therapy impossible. This protracted and difficult to control urticaria should not be confused with the appearance of acute and transient urticaria during desensitization, which is not uncommon.

In additional, during oral aspirin challenges, rare patients may experience significant gastrointestinal symptoms, with vomiting and epigastric pain. In this situation, starting an intravenous line may be useful. The authors have found that the use of sublingual or intravenous ondansetron, intravenous ranitidine, and oral Maalox can be helpful in controlling these symptoms. Pancreatitis has recently been reported in conjunction with aspirin desensitization as a cause-and-effect reaction.[28] Alternatively, aspirin may be an innocent bystander, particularly in the setting of biliary sludge and other less readily obvious causes of pancreatitis.[29] If aspirin caused pancreatitis, it must be exceeding rare and the mechanism for such a reaction is unknown. However, for any patients with symptoms resembling pancreatitis, an amylase and lipase test should be ordered. Laryngospasm can occur during OACs and actually may be underappreciated. Any symptoms, such as difficulty swallowing or dyspnea localized to the throat, should be treated with inhaled racemic epinephrine via nebulizer. A flow volume loop during spirometry may show acute blunting and notching of the inspiratory loop but the absence of this finding does not exclude intermittent vocal cord spasm. In fact, in patients with normal spirometry and significant dyspnea that does not respond to nebulized beta-agonists, a trial dose of inhaled racemic epinephrine should be considered.

As alluded to earlier, an unintended consequence of the use of montelukast and other leukotriene modifiers during desensitization is the outcome of "silent desensitization." Before the availability of montelukast in 1999, an OAC with no symptoms or changes in spirometry reliably identified a negative challenge and excluded a diagnosis of AERD. Silent desensitization was first documented in a study by Stevenson and colleagues[22] in 2000 and the authors are now aware of multiple patients who have had a negative OAC and then have gone on to have a second positive oral aspirin challenge, after montelukast was withdrawn.[30] Although it might not be feasible to perform a second definitive challenge after discontinuing montelukast, it should at least be considered particularly in those patients with a strong history of multiple recent NSAID-induced respiratory reactions. In a study at Scripps Clinic, looking back at historical asthmatic reactions to NSAIDs in a group of patients with 2 prior historical reactions to NSAIDs, 11% experienced negative OACs.[31] Because most patients were pretreated with montelukast, the authors' assumption is that in the 11% were some patients who underwent silent aspirin desensitization. This issue is more than academic. A patient with a false-negative challenge may assume or be counseled that they do not have AERD and do not need to worry about future NSAID-induced reactions. They are then denied the benefit of daily aspirin therapy and at risk of future reactions if montelukast is discontinued.

Aspirin desensitization should be the standard of care for patients with recalcitrant nasal polyposis, need for repeated sinus surgeries, significant systemic corticosteroid requirements, or an underlying medical condition requiring aspirin.[32] Nevertheless, it still is underused. Aside from concerns about safety, the other significant impediment to using aspirin desensitization is logistical factors, centering on the use of nursing staff, billing issues, and level of care necessary.

When considering costs, the authors have found that aspirin desensitization is routinely approved by most insurance plans. In fact, Shaker and colleagues[33] demonstrated that across a wide range of assumptions, aspirin desensitization was cost effective in AERD. Although there are certainly direct costs to the patient, such as time away from work (2–3 days), possibly an overnight hotel bill, and health plan deductibles or uncovered costs, these factors should be balanced against loss of work because of future sinus surgeries and costs associated with expensive medications and unintended physician or emergency visits. A true estimation of the burden of disease in AERD is difficult and must encompass asthma, chronic sinusitis, nasal polyposis, and an inability to take aspirin or NSAIDS.[34] The burden of disease is considerable when factoring in symptoms, medication requirements, multispecialty medical management, work absenteeism, and work presenteeism. Aspirin desensitization with ongoing aspirin therapy addresses and treats each component of the AERD tetrad, thus making it an ideal treatment option for these patients.

Recently in the United States, nasal ketorolac has been evaluated in a protocol that assists in the rapid accomplishment of acute aspirin desensitization.[35] This modified ketorolac oral aspirin challenge has been shown to be associated with less laryngospasm and gastrointestinal symptoms, which frequently delays aspirin desensitization. Thus, achieving aspirin desensitization has been reduced from an average of 3 days to 1.5 days (**Fig. 1**).

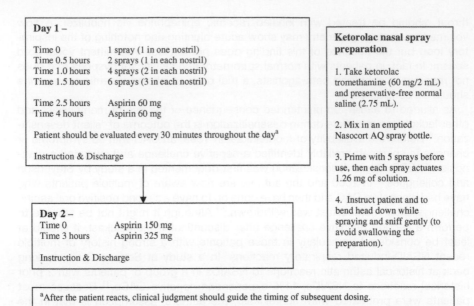

**Day 1 –**

| Time 0 | 1 spray (1 in one nostril) |
| Time 0.5 hours | 2 sprays (1 in each nostril) |
| Time 1.0 hours | 4 sprays (2 in each nostril) |
| Time 1.5 hours | 6 sprays (3 in each nostril) |
| Time 2.5 hours | Aspirin 60 mg |
| Time 4 hours | Aspirin 60 mg |

Patient should be evaluated every 30 minutes throughout the day[a]

Instruction & Discharge

**Ketorolac nasal spray preparation**

1. Take ketorolac tromethamine (60 mg/2 mL) and preservative-free normal saline (2.75 mL).

2. Mix in an emptied Nasocort AQ spray bottle.

3. Prime with 5 sprays before use, then each spray actuates 1.26 mg of solution.

4. Instruct patient and to bend head down while spraying and sniff gently (to avoid swallowing the preparation).

**Day 2 –**

| Time 0 | Aspirin 150 mg |
| Time 3 hours | Aspirin 325 mg |

Instruction & Discharge

[a]After the patient reacts, clinical judgment should guide the timing of subsequent dosing.

**Fig. 1.** Sample nasal Ketorolac and modified oral aspirin challenge.

There are several clinical aspects of aspirin desensitization and chronic aspirin therapy that warrant further consideration. Aspirin seems to be unique in its ability to modify the inflammatory components of AERD. As mentioned earlier, the dose of aspirin that is necessary for effectiveness is not the dose that would be necessary for antiplatelet-blocking or COX-1-blocking effects. Aspirin desensitization can be maintained with 81 mg aspirin per day. Although there are some patients who derive therapeutic benefit from aspirin 81 mg twice a day or 160 mg in the morning and 81 mg at night, this is unusual, and most patients are taking at least 325 mg twice a day. The authors' current practice is to start all patients on aspirin 650 mg twice a day for the first month, unless they have prior gastritis from NSAIDs or prior ulcer disease. After 1 month, if nasal passages are patent, a step down of aspirin to 650 mg in the morning and 325 mg at night, followed by 325 mg twice a day, is attempted. If a reappearance of nasal congestion occurs, aspirin dosages are increased in a stepwise fashion. Finally, and most paradoxically, is the finding that aspirin has no benefit in chronic sinus disease, with or without polyps, and asthma unless the patient has AERD. Understanding the mechanism of aspirin benefit may illuminate the answers to the pathogenesis of AERD in the first place and offer future targets for therapy.

**REFERENCES**

1. Widal F, Abrami P, Lermoyez J. Anaphylaxie et idiosyncrasie. La Presse Medicale 1922;30:189–93.
2. Klion AD. Widal on the aspirin triad and induction of tolerance. Allergy Proc 1993; 14:371–2.
3. Zeiss CR, Lockey RF. Refractory period to aspirin in a patient with aspirin-induced asthma. J Allergy Clin Immunol 1976;57:440–8.
4. Bianco S, Robushchi M, Petrigni G. Aspirin induced tolerance in aspirin-asthma detected by a new challenge test. IRCS J Med Sci 1977;5:129–36.

5. Pleskow WW, Stevenson DD, Mathison DA, et al. Aspirin desensitization in aspirin-sensitive asthmatic patients: clinical manifestations and characterization of the refractory period. J Allergy Clin Immunol 1982;69:11–9.
6. Stevenson DD, Simon RA, Mathison DA. Aspirin sensitive asthma: tolerance to aspirin after positive oral aspirin challenges. J Allergy Clin Immunol 1980;66: 82–8.
7. Lumry WR, Curd JG, Zeiger RS, et al. Aspirin-sensitive rhinosinusitis: the clinical syndrome and effects of aspirin administration. J Allergy Clin Immunol 1983;71: 580–7.
8. Stevenson DD, Pleskow WW, Simon RA, et al. Aspirin-sensitive rhinosinusitis asthma: a double-blind crossover study of treatment with aspirin. J Allergy Clin Immunol 1984;73:500–7.
9. Rozsasi A, Polzehl D, Deutschle T, et al. Long term treatment with aspirin desensitization: a prospective clinical trial comparing 100 and 300mg aspirin daily. Allergy 2008;63:1228–34.
10. Sweet JM, Stevenson DD, Simon RA, et al. Long-term effects of aspirin desensitization–treatment for aspirin-sensitive rhinosinusitis-asthma. J Allergy Clin Immunol 1990;85:59–65.
11. Stevenson DD, Hankammer MA, Mathison DA, et al. Aspirin desensitization treatment of aspirin-sensitive patients with rhinosinusitis-asthma: long-term outcomes. J Allergy Clin Immunol 1996;98:751–8.
12. Berges-Gimeno MP, Simon RA, Stevenson DD. Long-term treatment with aspirin desensitization in asthmatic patients with aspirin-exacerbated respiratory disease. J Allergy Clin Immunol 2003;111:180–6.
13. Lee JY, Simon RA, Stevenson DD. Selection of aspirin dosages for aspirin desensitization treatment with aspirin-exacerbated respiratory disease. J Allergy Clin Immunol 2007;119:157–64.
14. Kowalski ML, Grzelewska-Rzymowska I, Szmidt M. Clinical efficacy of aspirin in "desensitized" aspirin-sensitive asthmatics. Eur J Respir Dis 1986;69:219–25.
15. Berges-Gimeno MP, Simon RA, Stevenson DD. Early effects of aspirin desensitization treatment in asthmatic patients with aspirin-exacerbated respiratory disease. Ann Allergy Asthma Immunol 2003;90:338–41.
16. Stevenson DD, Simon RA. Respiratory sensitivity: respiratory and cutaneous manifestations. In: Middleton E Jr, Reed CE, Ellis EF, et al, editors. Allergy principles and practice, vol. 3. St Louis (MO): CV Mosby Co; 1988. p. 1541.
17. Szczeklik A, Serwonska M. Inhibition of idiosyncratic reactions to aspirin in asthmatic patients by clemastine. Thorax 1979;34:654–7.
18. Sladek K, Szczeklik A. Cysteinyl leukotrienes overproduction and mast cell activation in aspirin-provoked bronchospasm in asthma. Eur Respir J 1993;6:391–9.
19. Daffern PJ, Muilenburg D, Stevenson DD, et al. Association of urinary leukotriene E4 excretion during aspirin challenges with severity of respiratory responses. J Allergy Clin Immunol 1999;1:559–64.
20. Berges-Gimeno MP, Simon RA, Stevenson DD. The effect of leukotriene-modifier drugs on aspirin-induced asthma and rhinitis reactions. Clin Exp Allergy 2002;32: 1491–6.
21. White AA, Stevenson DD, Simon RA, et al. The blocking effect of essential controller medications during aspirin challenges in patients with aspirin-exacerbated respiratory disease. Ann Allergy Asthma Immunol 2005;95:330–5.
22. Stevenson DD, Simon RA, Mathison DA, et al. Montelukast is only partially effective in inhibiting aspirin responses in aspirin-sensitive asthmatics. Ann Allergy Asthma Immunol 2000;85:477–82.

23. White A, Ludington E, Mehra P, et al. Effect of leukotriene modifier drugs on the safety of oral aspirin challenges. Ann Allergy Asthma Immunol 2006;97:688–93.

24. Williams AN, Simon RA, Woessner KM, et al. The relationship between historical aspirin-induced asthma and severity of asthma induced during oral aspirin challenges. J Allergy Clin Immunol 2007;120:273–7.

25. Hope AP, Woessner KA, Simon RA, et al. Rational approach to aspirin dosing during oral challenges and desensitization of patients with aspirin-exacerbated respiratory disease. J Allergy Clin Immunol 2009;123:406–10.

26. White AA, Hope AP, Stevenson DD. Failure to maintain an aspirin-desensitized state in a patient with aspirin-exacerbated respiratory disease. Ann Allergy Asthma Immunol 2006;97:446–8.

27. Simon RA. Prevention and treatment of reactions to NSAIDs. Clin Rev Allergy Immunol 2003;24:189–98.

28. Hoyte FC, Weber RW, Katial RK. Pancreatitis as a novel complication of aspirin therapy in patients with aspirin exacerbated respiratory disease. J Allergy Clin Immunol 2012;129:1684–6.

29. Stevenson DD, White AA, Simon RA. Aspirin as a cause of pancreatitis in patients with aspirin-exacerbated respiratory disease. J Allergy Clin Immunol 2012;129: 1687–8.

30. White AA, Bosso JV, Stevenson DD. The clinical dilemma of "silent desensitization" in aspirin exacerbated respiratory disease. Allergy Asthma Proc, in press.

31. Dursun AB, Woessner KA, Simon RA, et al. Predicting outcomes of oral aspirin challenges in patients with asthma, nasal polyps, and chronic sinusitis. Ann Allergy Asthma Immunol 2008;100:420–5.

32. Stevenson DD, Simon RA. Selection of patients for aspirin desensitization treatment. J Allergy Clin Immunol 2006;118:801–4.

33. Shaker M, Lobb A, Jenkins P, et al. An economic analysis of aspirin desensitization in aspirin-exacerbated respiratory disease. J Allergy Clin Immunol 2008;121: 81–7.

34. Chang JE, White AA, Simon RA, et al. Aspirin-exacerbated respiratory disease: burden of disease. Allergy Asthma Proc 2012;33(2):117–21.

35. Lee RU, White AA, Ding D, et al. Use of intranasal ketorolac and modified oral aspirin challenge for desensitization of aspirin-exacerbated respiratory disease. Ann Allergy Asthma Immunol 2010;105:130–5.

# Mechanisms of Aspirin Desensitization

Trever Burnett, MD[a], Rohit Katial, MD[b],*, Rafeul Alam, MD, PhD[c]

## KEYWORDS

- Aspirin-exacerbated respiratory disease (AERD) • Aspirin desensitization
- Mechanisms of action • Cysteinyl leukotrienes (CysLTs) • Cytokines
- Interleukin 4 (IL-4) • Signal transducer and activator of transcription 6 (STAT6)

## KEY POINTS

- Aspirin-exacerbated respiratory disease (AERD) is characterized by severe, persistent asthma, hyperplastic eosinophilic sinusitis with nasal polyps, and intolerance to aspirin and other nonsteroidal antiinflammatory drugs.
- Aspirin desensitization is an effective therapeutic option in carefully selected patients.
- AERD is associated with an overexpression of cysteinyl leukotrienes (CysLTs), with marked upregulation of CysLT receptors.
- Despite increased knowledge about the pathophysiology underlying AERD, the mechanisms behind the therapeutic effects of aspirin desensitization remain poorly understood.
- Recent studies suggest that the clinical benefits of aspirin desensitization may occur through direct inhibition of tyrosine kinases and the signal transducer and activator of transcription 6 pathway, with resultant inhibition of interleukin 4 production.

## INTRODUCTION

It has been almost 100 years since Widal[1] first described aspirin (acetylsalicylic acid) challenges and desensitization for patients with the syndrome of asthma, nasal polyposis, and aspirin intolerance. Later, after works by Samter and Beers, the condition was termed Samter triad because of the association of these 3 overlapping

Funding Sources: Dr Burnett, Dr Katial: None. Dr Alam: National Institutes of Health.
Conflict of Interest: None.
[a] Adult Program, Department of Allergy and Immunology, National Jewish Medical and Research Center, University of Colorado, 1400 Jackson Street, K624, Denver, CO 80206, USA;
[b] Weinberg Clinical Research Unit, Adult Fellowship Program, Department of Allergy and Immunology, National Jewish Medical and Research Center, University of Colorado, 1400 Jackson Street, K624, Denver, CO 80206, USA; [c] Division of Allergy and Immunology, National Jewish Medical and Research Center, University of Colorado, 1400 Jackson Street, K624, Denver, CO 80206, USA
* Corresponding author.
E-mail address: KatialR@NJHealth.org

conditions.[2] As discussed elsewhere in this issue, it has since been called by many terms, including aspirin-sensitive asthma, aspirin-intolerant asthma, and aspirin idiosyncrasy, although in most of the world, aspirin-exacerbated respiratory disease (AERD) is now the preferred nomenclature. In a double-blind, crossover study published in 1984 by Stevenson and colleagues,[3] aspirin desensitization therapy was shown to provide significant clinical improvement in nasal symptoms and requirement for nasal steroids. Symptom improvement has been reported to occur as early as 4 weeks after initiation of aspirin therapy, and long-term benefits include significant reductions in the number of sinus infections and operations, hospitalizations for asthma, and use of systemic steroids.[4,5] Despite these data, which support the clinical benefit, the mechanisms of aspirin therapy are still not clearly understood.

Published data suggest that the disease occurs because of chronic inflammation resulting from an imbalance of endogenous inflammatory and antiinflammatory mediators produced from the metabolism of arachidonic acid (also known as eicosatetraenoic acid).[6] Abnormalities in these eicosanoid mediators (including leukotrienes [LTs], prostaglandins [PGs], lipoxins [LXs] and their respective receptors) have all been implicated in the pathogenesis of AERD.[7] The cysteinyl LTs (CysLTs) (LTC$_4$, LTD$_4$, and LTE$_4$), which are metabolized from arachidonic acid via the 5-lipoxygenase pathway are powerful mediators of airway hyperresponsiveness, vascular permeability, bronchoconstriction, collagen deposition, and eosinophil chemotaxis and activation.[8] Evidence reveals that baseline expression of CysLTs is increased in patients with AERD and these levels further increase in response to specific aspirin challenge.[9–15] This situation may be caused by the increased expression of LTC$_4$ synthase (LTC$_4$S) seen in tissue mast cells (MC) and eosinophils of patients with AERD when compared with aspirin-tolerant asthmatics (ATAs).[16,17] In addition, patients with AERD show upregulation of the CysLT$_1$ receptors and an underexpression of the counterregulatory PGE$_2$ receptors when compared with ATAs.[18,19] Recent studies suggest that the AERD phenotype may result from an overproduction of the cytokine interleukin 4 (IL-4).[20–23] Aspirin desensitization and continued therapy results in reduced urinary LTE$_4$ (uLTE$_4$) levels and CysLT$_1$ receptor expression, which may occur through direct inhibition of the IL-4–activated signal transducer and activator of transcription 6 (STAT6) pathway.[20,23–25] These findings give insight into the mechanism of aspirin desensitization and are the subject of this review.

## ASPIRIN AND NONSTEROIDAL ANTIINFLAMMATORY DRUG PHARMACOLOGY

Aspirin was first synthesized by Felix Hoffman in 1897 and was marketed by Bayer as an antiinflammatory drug.[26] The mechanism of action was not determined until 1971, when John Vane published his Nobel prize-winning discovery that aspirin and other nonsteroidal antiinflammatory drug (NSAID) medications inhibited PG production.[27] There are now more than 20 commercially available NSAIDs, which are all absorbed completely, have minimal first-pass metabolism, are tightly bound to albumin, and have small volumes of distribution.[28,29]

Aspirin and NSAIDs induce PG inhibition through binding and inactivation of cyclooxygenase (COX), also known as PG endoperoxide synthase.[26] COX exists in 2 isoforms (COX-1 and COX-2), which convert arachidonic acid to PGH$_2$ which is then rapidly converted to the bioactive prostanoids PGE$_2$ and thromboxane A$_2$.[30] The COX-1 and COX-2 structures are about 60% homologous, and both isoforms have a molecular weight of about 71 kDa.[27] The COX active site is a long, hydrophobic channel, which aspirin enters and then causes irreversible inhibition by acetylation of serine 529 residue in COX-1 and serine 516 in COX-2.[31] However, the active site of COX-2 is slightly larger than the active site of COX-1, which allows for the selectivity of specific COX-2 inhibitors, which are too large to inactivate COX-1 enzymes.[26] In addition, this size difference permits some continued activity of COX-2 despite aspirin binding, which allows the conversion of arachidonic acid to 15R-hydroxyeicosatetraenoic acid (15R-HETE) in the LX pathway, producing powerful antiinflammatory mediators.[27] COX-1 is constitutively expressed and performs housekeeping functions, producing PGs that regulate normal cell activity. The concentration of the COX-1 enzyme remains generally stable, although it can increase in response to some stimuli, hormones, or growth factors.[30] Concentrations of COX-2 are minimal in resting cells but can be induced by inflammatory stimuli. Recently, a COX-3 isoform has also been identified that is inhibited by paracetamol (acetaminophen) and low concentrations of aspirin and other NSAIDs.[26]

## DESENSITIZATION EFFECTS ON PRODUCTS OF ARACHIDONIC ACID METABOLISM

Aspirin desensitization results in both acute and chronic changes in the expression and production of arachidonic acid mediators and their respective receptors. However, the alterations in some of these mediators (PG, LT, and LX) alone cannot account for all of the clinical benefits of aspirin therapy.[5] LTE$_4$ is the most stable of the CysLTs and mediates many of the principal aspects of AERD, including bronchial constriction, hyperresponsiveness, eosinophilia, and increased vascular permeability.[32] As mentioned earlier, uLTE$_4$ excretion is increased in patients with AERD both at baseline and after aspirin administration, and the intensity of the reaction to aspirin challenge correlates with the degree of baseline increase.[19] This correlation between increased uLTE$_4$ levels in patients with a more severe response to aspirin challenge is not surprising given that LTE$_4$ administered via inhalational challenge induces severe bronchial constriction.[33] Although these studies prove LTE$_4$ to be a significant mediator of disease in patients with AERD, the severe inflammatory response is inconsistent with the relative low affinity of LTE$_4$ for the CysLT$_1$ and CysLT$_2$ receptors.[8] This contradiction suggests the possibility of an alternative, more specific CysLT$_E$R through which LTE$_4$ signaling is mediated. The alternative receptor hypothesis is further supported by evidence published by Maekawa and colleagues,[34] who reported that significant vascular leak persists after LTE$_4$ intradermal injections, even in CysLT$_1$R/CysLT$_2$R double-deficient mice. Although a specific CysLT$_E$R has yet to be identified, one possibility may be the adenosine diphosphate-reactive purinergic (P2Y$_{12}$) receptor, which is required for LTE$_4$-potentiated airway inflammation in mice.[35] These findings need to be further explored in humans and more specifically in patients with AERD.

Nasser and colleagues[36] studied the effects of aspirin desensitization on uLTE$_4$ concentrations in 9 patients with AERD. uLTE$_4$ levels were measured before and then at specific time intervals for 9 hours after aspirin administration. Comparison was made between (1) an initial dose of aspirin (mean of approximately 90 mg), which resulted in a 15% reduction in FEV$_1$ (forced expiratory volume in first second of expiration); (2) 600 mg aspirin 24 hours after desensitization; and (3) the 600-mg maintenance dose at least 2 months after desensitization. The initial dose of aspirin resulted in a 7-fold increase in uLTE$_4$ from baseline levels at 3 hours after ingestion. The comparable increases were 3-fold after initial desensitization and 2-fold with maintenance aspirin dosing (**Fig. 1**). Overall, the uLTE4 production was reduced by 82% and 86% after initial desensitization and with continued maintenance therapy, respectively. The maximum reduction in FEV$_1$ was also improved from 15.3% $\pm$ 3.9% after initial aspirin dosing, to 3.3% $\pm$ 2.4% after initial desensitization and

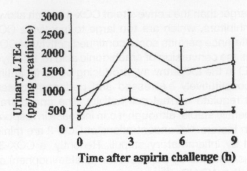

**Fig. 1.** uLTE₄ levels in 5 patients for 9 hours after challenge at the threshold dose of aspirin (○) and with 600 mg aspirin at 24 hours (△) and at 9 (3.2) months after aspirin desensitization (●). Each point is mean ± standard error of the mean. (*Reprinted from* Nasser S, Patel M, Bell G, et al. The effect of aspirin desensitization on urinary leukotriene E4 concentrations in aspirin-sensitive asthma. Am J Respir Crit Care Med 1995;151:1329; with permission.)

7.4% ± 4.5% with continued therapy (**Fig. 2**). Additional studies also showed that continued aspirin therapy after successful desensitization results in a 20-fold reduction in bronchial responsiveness to inhaled LTE₄.[37] Together these findings show that in patients with AERD, aspirin desensitization results in both decreased production of LTE₄ and reduced airway responsiveness to LTE₄. The mechanisms of these changes have not been identified.

LTB₄, which is metabolized from LTA₄ via LTA₄ hydrolase, is a potent chemotactic factor for eosinophils and neutrophils and contributes to the chronic inflammation seen in AERD.[6] Juergens and colleagues[38] studied the release of LTB₄ and LTC₄ from calcium ionophore-stimulated peripheral blood monocytes from patients with AERD and normal volunteers before and after acute desensitization. Consistent with previous studies, patients with AERD had increased baseline levels of TXB₂, LTB₄, and LTC₄. After aspirin desensitization, TXB₂ was almost completely suppressed in both groups.

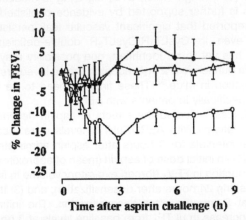

**Fig. 2.** Percent change in FEV₁ in 5 patients for 9 hours after challenge at the threshold dose of aspirin (○) and with 600 mg aspirin at 24 hours (△) and at 9 (3.2) months after aspirin desensitization (●). Each point is mean ± standard error of the mean. (*Reprinted from* Nasser S, Patel M, Bell G, et al. The effect of aspirin desensitization on urinary leukotriene E4 concentrations in aspirin-sensitive asthma. Am J Respir Crit Care Med 1995;151:1328; with permission.)

$LTB_4$ release was reduced by 42% in the group of patients with AERD. $LTC_4$ levels were also increased at baseline and decreased after desensitization; however, the changes were not significant. Clinically, 8 of the 10 patients with AERD were taking prednisone before aspirin challenge. After desensitization, prednisone dosing was reduced, with an 85% reduction in average steroid dose (10.4 ± 2.2 mg/d to 1.6 ± 2.8 mg/d). This clinical change may have resulted from the decreased $LTB_4$ production, with a subsequent reduction in chemotactic-mediated tissue inflammation.

LXs are generated from arachidonic acid via sequential action of 2 or more lipoxygenases.[39] They are generally formed as a product of cell-cell interactions via transcellular biosynthetic routes that occur during tissue inflammation and disease pathogenesis.[40] These substances have important antiinflammatory effects, reducing cellular influx into inflammatory sites and competing for CysLT receptors, thus inhibiting CysLT-associated responses.[41] Nasal polyp tissue has a high capacity to produce LXs.[42] However, research reveals that compared with ATAs, patients with AERD have impaired whole blood $LXA_4$ production even when exposed to IL-3 or cationic ionophore activation.[43] The aspirin-sensitive patients also had reduced 15-epi-LXA4, which is produced via COX-2 in the presence of aspirin. Additional studies have revealed that COX-2 remains active after aspirin acetylation and is able to convert arachidonic acid substrates into the R-enantiomer of 15R-HETE.[44] This R-enantiomer is further metabolized to 15-epi-$LXA_4$, which is more potent and longer-acting than its native 15S form because of less rapid metabolic inactivation.[40] This aspirin-triggered LT (ATL) analogue inhibits the phosphorylation of leukocyte-specific protein 1 via the p38–mitogen-activated protein (MAP) kinase pathway, which is important in the activation, chemotaxis, and other proinflammatory responses of neutrophils.[45] Such antiinflammatory mechanisms may play a part in the routine health and cardioprotective benefits seen in nonasthmatic patients who have increased ATL levels even on low-dose daily aspirin therapy.[46] However, production of these LX and ATL analogues is dependent on COX-2 enzyme expression. which has been shown to be reduced in patients with AERD with chronic rhinosinusitis (CRS) when compared with aspirin-tolerant and normal adult patients.[39] Although reduced COX-2 expression accounts for the baseline reduced LX levels in patients with AERD, there have still been no studies looking at the long-term changes in LX and ATL analogue generation that may occur after successful aspirin desensitization. It is hoped that further investigation will highlight some of the therapeutic benefits and mechanisms behind aspirin desensitization.

## DESENSITIZATION EFFECTS ON CYSLT RECEPTOR EXPRESSION

CysLT receptors have been divided into mainly 2 classes ($CysLT_1R$ and $CysLT_2R$), although additional receptor isoforms have been proposed.[8] There is only about 38% homology between these 2 receptors, accounting for their varied sensitivities for each of the CysLT ($CysLT_1R$ – $LTD_4 \gg LTC_4 > LTE_4$; $CysLT_2R$ – $LTD_4 = LTC_4 > LTE_4$). $CysLT_1R$ is expressed in the spleen, lung, and smooth muscle, whereas $CysLT_2R$ has greater expression in the heart, pulmonary vein, adrenal medulla, and placenta. Studies have also revealed the presence of $CysLT_1R$ on peripheral blood leukocytes.[47] Both receptors are recognized as membrane-bound G-protein-coupled receptors, and signaling occurs through activation of an MAP kinase response pathway.[47] The receptors are regulated immunologically by several cytokines. $CysLT_1R$ expression can be upregulated in human monocytes and macrophages by exposure to the Th2 cytokines IL-4, IL-5, and IL-13. $CysLT_2R$ expression is upregulated by the Th2 cytokine IL-4 in human umbilical vein endothelial cells. Interferon

$\gamma$ (IFN-$\gamma$) is able to induce expression of both receptors in airway smooth muscle cells. Tumor necrosis factor $\alpha$ (TNF-$\alpha$) and IL-1$\beta$ tend to be counterregulatory.[8]

CRS with nasal polyposis is a characteristic feature of AERD, as discussed elsewhere in this issue. Abnormalities in local arachidonic acid metabolism in these patients include low production of PGE$_2$, high release of CysLTs, and downregulation of COX-2 enzyme.[48] In 2002, Sousa and colleagues[18] examined the expression of CysLT$_1$ and LTB$_4$ receptors in inflammatory leukocytes from nasal biopsies of patients with AERD. Specimens were obtained from 22 aspirin-sensitive patients and 12 aspirin-tolerant controls. Eighteen of the 22 aspirin-sensitive patients underwent a randomized, double-blind, placebo-controlled trial of topical desensitization with intranasal lysine aspirin. Results showed that baseline CysLT$_1$R expression was significantly higher in cells from patients with AERD compared with non–aspirin-sensitive controls (median, 542 cells/mm$^2$ [range, 148–1390] vs 116 cells/mm$^2$ [range, 40–259]; $P<.001$). There was no difference in LTB$_4$ receptor expression. Desensitization was associated with a significant reduction in cells expressing the CysLT$_1$R, which was seen as early as 2 weeks and persisted through follow-up at 6 months. Though this finding may partially explain the clinical benefit of aspirin desensitization, the study did not postulate further as to why the CysLT$_1$R were downregulated with continued aspirin therapy. As is discussed in the following section, this downregulation likely results from aspirin-induced changes in IL-4 production.

## IL-4 ALTERATIONS AFTER ASPIRIN DESENSITIZATION

The cascade of inflammation in AERD involves the stimulatory signaling of various cytokines. Specific associations may include IL-5 promotion of eosinophil development, differentiation, and survival, and IL-13–enhanced bronchial smooth muscle proliferation and inhibition of PGE$_2$ biosynthesis.[6] More recently, research has focused on the role of IL-4 in the development of AERD. IL-4 is produced by T$_H$2-type helper T cells, MC, basophils, and activated eosinophils.[49] It has regulatory functions in the production of IgE by B lymphocytes and stimulatory effects on epithelial cell mucous hypersecretion and collagen production by fibroblasts. Hsieh and colleagues[50] studied the priming effects of IL-4 on the production of histamine, CysLTs, and PGs from human MC derived in vitro from cord blood mononuclear cells. CysLT release was increased by 27-fold and PGD$_2$ release was increased by 6-fold when these MC were passively stimulated with IL-4 in addition to stem cell factor (SCF). CysLT production was further increased 6-fold and 4-fold by the addition of IL-3 or IL-5, respectively, to the IL-4/SCF-primed cells. This increase was found to occur as a result of increased IL-4 induction of LTC$_4$S. Additional evidence published by Early and colleagues[51] shows the compounded effects of IL-4 on CysLT receptor expression. Using quantitative polymerase chain reaction analysis of mRNA and receptor proteins extracted from immune cells, the investigators were able to show that IL-4 stimulation resulted in significant increases in both CysLT$_1$R and CysLT$_2$R on T and B lymphocytes ($P<.01$) and CysLT$_2$R only on eosinophils ($P<.05$). CysLT$_2$R mRNA was also increased in monoctyes, T cells, and B cells after IFN-$\gamma$ stimulation. The mechanisms of these effects have been shown to occur through IL-4/STAT6-dependent pathways, which are also important in the IL-4–induced suppression of PG production.[52–54] Combined results from these studies imply a likely role for IL-4 in the pathogenesis of AERD.

The pharmacologic effects of aspirin beyond COX-related inhibition have been extended to include the inhibition of IL-4. Cianferoni and colleagues[24] examined the effect of aspirin on the expression of various cytokines, including IL-4, IL13, IL-2, and IFN-γ in purified human CD4⁺ T cells. Experiments showed that therapeutic concentrations of aspirin significantly inhibited IL-4 secretion in peripheral blood T cells by 47% ± 2.4% (P<.05) and that this inhibition occurred without significant aspirin-induced apoptosis to account for the change. Using multiple NSAIDs, the investigators showed that IL-4 suppression occurred independently of COX inhibition. They identified aspirin inhibition of IL-4 gene expression via salicylate-targeted regions in the IL-4 promoter as the possible mechanism of action, although the exact pathway was not defined. Aspirin did not have any significant affect on the levels of IL-2, IL-13, or IFN-γ expression.

Expanding on these findings, several groups have now identified aspirin inhibition of IL-4–induced STAT6 activation as the possible mechanism associated with the therapeutic benefits of aspirin desensitization. Using a murine model, Perez-G and colleagues[55] showed that sodium salicylate (NaSal) and aspirin blocked the ability of IL-4 to induce DNA-binding activity of STAT6 in a dose-dependent manner (**Fig. 3**). They showed that aspirin inhibits IL-4–dependent induction of CD23 expression on human peripheral blood mononuclear cells and that both of these results were dependent on Src family kinases, which were blocked by aspirin. These findings were confirmed in a more recent study published by Steinke and colleagues.[25] Using THP-1 human mononuclear cells, they showed that aspirin inhibited IL-4–induced CysLT$_1$R and F$_{cε}$RI$_α$ mRNA expression in a dose-dependent fashion. Similar results occurred with ketorolac but not NaSal. These investigators also reported the presence of STAT6-binding sites within the promoters for the CysLT$_1$R and LTC$_4$S, which are engaged by IL-4 nuclear extracts and were effectively inhibited by aspirin.

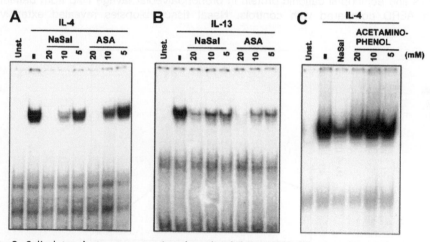

**Fig. 3.** Salicylates, but not acetaminophenol, inhibit STAT6 activation. (*A*) M12 cells were cultured with the indicated concentrations of NaSal and aspirin for 1 hour before stimulation with IL-4 (10 ng/mL) for 30 minutes. STAT6 DNA-binding activity in cell extracts was analyzed by electrophoretic mobility shift assay (EMSA) using the IFN-γ activation site sequence contained in the Cε promoter. (*B*) U937 cells were cultured with NaSal or ASA for 1 hour, and then stimulated for 30 minutes with IL-13 (400 ng/mL). STAT6 activation was then analyzed by EMSA. (*C*) M12 cells were cultured with nothing, NaSal (20 mM), or the indicated concentrations of acetaminophenol. IL-4 was then added, and STAT6 binding to DNA was analyzed by EMSA. (*Reprinted from* Perez-GM, Melo M, Keegan A, et al. Aspirin and salicylates inhibit the IL-4 and IL-13 induced activation of STAT6. J Immunol 2002;168:1429; with permission.)

Katial and colleagues[20] reported the effects of aspirin desensitization on novel inflammatory sputum biomarkers in patients with AERD. In addition to IL-4, these investigators studied changes in sputum tryptase, matrix metallopeptidase 9 (MMP-9), tissue inhibitors of metalloproteinases 1 (TIMP-1) and FMS-like tyrosine kinase 3 ligand. Traditional measures such as symptoms scores, exhaled nitric oxide (FeNO), and lung function were also assessed. Twenty-one patients were enrolled in the study, with 16 completing successful sputum induction. Symptom scores were significantly improved after 6 months of aspirin therapy, comparable with previous studies. FeNO levels increased more than baseline by 20% ($P = .03$) during the acute desensitization and remained more than baseline after 6 months, although the difference was not significant. Positive correlations were seen between MMP-9 and TIMP-1 and MMP-9 and tryptase, all of which were increased immediately after desensitization. At 6 months after desensitization, sputum IL-4 levels decreased 94.7% (95% confidence interval [CI], 67%–99.2%) relative to baseline (baseline mean 28.1 pg/mL, 6-month mean 1.5 pg/mL; $P = .004$) (**Fig. 4**). This change was accompanied with a similar decrease in MMP-9 after 6 months. These findings suggest that the reported increases in CysLTs and their receptors are regulated by IL-4–dependent pathways, which are then downregulated by daily aspirin treatment after desensitization.

## EOSINOPHIL AND MC RESPONSES AFTER DESENSITIZATION

Data regarding inflammatory cell populations from both direct and indirect observations have identified MC and eosinophils as the primary infiltrating cells in patients with AERD. As previously discussed, Sladek and colleagues[13] found increased eosinophils and eosinophil cationic protein in bronchoalveolar lavage fluid from patients with AERD compared with controls. Nasal tissue biopsies revealed extensive

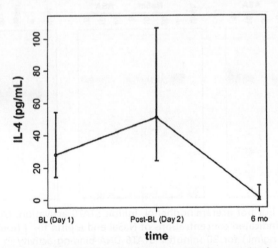

**Fig. 4.** IL-4 means over time, with 95% CIs, based on the linear mixed model fit. IL-4 was modeled on the natural log scale, and estimated and CI end points were then inverted back for presentation, resulting in longer upper bars than lower bars. Note that CIs are relevant for fixed time points only and do not indicate variability of estimated for differences between time points because repeated-measures data were involved. BL, baseline. (*Reprinted from* Katial R, Strand M, Prasertsuntarasai T, et al. The effect of aspirin desensitization on novel biomarkers in aspirin-exacerbated respiratory diseases. J Allergy Clin Immunol 2010;126:741; with permission.)

infiltration of eosinophils and degranulated MC.[56] In addition, nasal washes from patients with AERD after nasal aspirin-lysine challenge have shown significantly increased numbers of eosinophils when compared with controls.[57] Nasser and colleagues[16] obtained bronchial biopsies from 12 patients with AERD who had significantly increased MC and eosinophils but fewer numbers of macrophages when compared with aspirin-tolerant controls. The same investigators also completed a series of bronchial biopsies before and after endobronchial instillation of aspirin-lysine in 7 patients with AERD. Biopsies were separated by 20 minutes, and compared with baseline, specimens had decreased MC and increased activated eosinophils. These investigators postulated that these findings were a result of cell degranulation after aspirin dosing.[58] The only long-term data on cellular changes are extrapolated from the article by Sousa and colleagues,[18] which showed no changes in the numbers of CD45+ leukocytes between baseline and 2 weeks or 6 months after desensitization. These investigators did not report any data regarding changes in eosinophil or MC numbers.

There are limited data regarding what happens to eosinophil and MC inflammatory mediators with continued aspirin therapy. Bosso and colleagues[59] reported increased serum histamine and tryptase release in 3 patients after single-blinded oral aspirin challenge complicated by moderate to severe respiratory reactions with extended skin or gastrointestinal symptoms. However, in the other 14 patients who experienced similar pulmonary reactions but with no extrapulmonary manifestations, changes in histamine and tryptase were not observed. In a separate study, 8 patients with AERD were found to have increased symptoms, tryptase, histamine, and CysLT levels after oral aspirin challenge.[60] These effects were not altered by zileuton administration during a repeat challenge 2 weeks after initial testing.

## ALTERNATIVE ANTIINFLAMMATORY EFFECTS OF ASPIRIN THERAPY

Aspirin has numerous antiinflammatory effects related to both its COX inhibition as well as alternative mechanisms, which are currently being defined. The benefits of these effects are being exploited in numerous conditions, including cardiovascular diseases and cancer prevention, and there is speculation that aspirin can prevent new-onset asthma in adult patients.[61] The mechanisms range from increased LX production to inhibition of various intracellular signaling and nuclear transcription pathways. Although not all of these mechanisms have specific correlation in patients with AERD, they do provide insight into possible areas of future investigation.

In 1994, Kopp and Ghosh[62] published data on NSAID effects on nuclear transcription factor NF-κβ. They investigated the effects of NaSal and aspirin on the lipopolysaccharide (LPS)-induced NF-κβ activation in human Jurkat T-cell and the mouse pre–B-cell lines (PD31). NF-κβ is an inducible transcription factor that is bound in the cytoplasm to an inhibitor protein Iκβ. It is activated by stimulants including bacterial LPS, double-stranded RNA, IL-1, and TNF-α. It is then released from Iκβ and enters the nucleus, where it regulates transcription of specific genes involved in immune and inflammatory responses. The investigators found that aspirin and NaSal inhibit NF-κβ activation by preventing Iκβ phosphorylation or degradation in the cytoplasm. In a later study by Yin and colleagues,[63] this inhibition was reported to occur through specific inhibition by aspirin and NaSal of Iκκ-β, 1 of 2 kinases (the other is Iκκ-α) that phosphorylate Iκβ, leading to its degradation and subsequent release of NF-κβ. Other investigators have reported that NaSal inhibits TNF-induced activation of Iκβα phosphorylation and degradation in a p38-MAP kinase-dependent pathway.[64] In AERD, these pathways have not been specifically defined as contributing to the disease

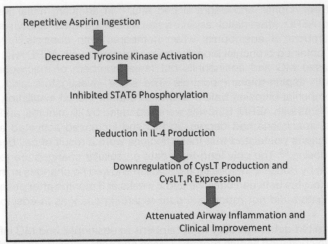

**Fig. 5.** Mechanism of inhibition of inflammation after aspirin desensitization. Proposed cascade of events after aspirin desensitization and continued ingestion. Signal inhibition via an IL-4/STAT6 pathway results in downregulation of CysLT production and CysLT$_1$R expression, with subsequent reduction of tissue inflammation.

process. Cianferoni and colleagues,[24] in their study on aspirin inhibition of IL-4 in human T cells, looked at NF-κβ as a possible link between the 2, but found no association.

NFAT is another nuclear transcription factor that is involved in the regulation of immune and inflammatory responses. Aceves and colleagues[65] attempted to examine the possible effects of salicylates on NFAT activation. Using aspirin and a trifluoromethylated salicylate derivative (triflusal), they were able to show a dose-dependent inhibition of several NFAT-regulated cytokine genes, including IL-2, IL-3, IL-8, GM-CSF, TNF-α, IFN-γ, and TGF-β1. Consistent with the other data we have reviewed, inhibition occurred only at higher therapeutic concentrations than used to inhibit COX. The medications also inhibited NFAT-dependent transcription, although triflusal was found to be the most potent. Mechanisms were determined to occur through possible inhibition of NFAT binding to DNA and NFAT transactivation. Thus, it acts differently from cyclosporin A, which inhibits calcineurin-induced dephosphorylation of NFAT, preventing its translocation to the nucleus. Additional mechanisms of aspirin activity include inhibition of activator protein 1, activation of adenosine monophosphate-activated protein kinase, and inhibition of the mechanistic target of rapamycin, which may be important in the benefit of aspirin in colorectal cancer.[66–68] Further research is needed to determine if any of these mechanistic pathways play a role in either the development of AERD or the benefit seen with daily aspirin treatment after desensitization.

## SUMMARY

AERD is a clinical syndrome characterized by severe, persistent asthma, hyperplastic eosinophilic sinusitis with nasal polyps, and an intolerance to aspirin and other NSAIDs that preferentially inhibit COX-1. The disease is associated with increased tissue infiltration by MC and eosinophils, overexpression of proinflammatory CysLTs, along with upregulation of CysLT$_1$ receptors. Aspirin or COX-1 inhibiting NSAID ingestion results in an acute reaction characterized by a reduction in PGs, including $PGE_2$, and a subsequent increase in CysLT production. Although aspirin desensitization has proved to be of significant long-term benefit in carefully selected patients with AERD, the mechanisms behind the therapeutic effects of aspirin desensitization remain poorly understood. Current research suggests that the derangements in inflammatory mediators seen in AERD may in part be a result of increased production and hyperresponsiveness to IL-4. This suggestion is reinforced by evidence that aspirin may derive its therapeutic benefit through direct inhibition of the IL-4–activated STAT6 pathway. The proposed mechanism would occur from continued aspirin ingestion causing inhibition of IL-4/STAT6–mediated production of CysLT and $CysLT_1R$ expression, with a subsequent attenuation of airway inflammation and clinical improvement (**Fig. 5**).

Despite these advances, the limited data published regarding long-term mechanistic effects after aspirin desensitization leave many outstanding questions: what is the molecular mechanism of aspirin desensitization? How does aspirin inhibit tyrosine kinases? What is the effect of aspirin on other cytokines? How many different cell types are targeted by aspirin desensitization? What is the effect of aspirin desensitization on the $LTE_4$-specific purinergic $P2Y_{12}$ receptor? Answering these questions requires further prospective, long-term evaluations of both the cellular and signaling alterations that occur in patients undergoing desensitization. In addition, as we learn more about the varied mechanisms of aspirin therapy related to inhibition of nuclear transcription factors, we may define new avenues of research exploration. Such further investigation will continue to increase our insight and understanding of this complex disease and it is hoped provide new therapeutic options and treatments for our patients.

## REFERENCES

1. Widal M, Abrami P, Lermeyez J. Anaphylaxieetidiosyncrasie. Presse Med 1922; 30:189–92.
2. Samter M, Beers R. Intolerance to aspirin: clinical studies and consideration of its pathogenesis. Ann Intern Med 1968;68:975–83.
3. Stevenson D, Pleskow W, Simon R, et al. Aspirin-sensitive rhinosinusitis asthma: a double-blind cross-over study of treatment with aspirin. J Allergy Clin Immunol 1984;73:500–7.
4. Berges-Gimeno M, Simon R, Stevenson D. Early effects of aspirin desensitization treatment in asthmatic patients with aspirin-exacerbated respiratory disease. Ann Allergy Asthma Immunol 2003;90:338–41.
5. Berges-Gimeno M, Simon R, Stevenson D. Long-term treatment with aspirin desensitization in asthmatic patients with aspirin-exacerbated respiratory disease. J Allergy Clin Immunol 2003;111:180–6.
6. Farooque S, Lee T. Aspirin-sensitive respiratory disease. Annu Rev Physiol 2009; 71:465–87.
7. Szczeklik A, Stevenson D. Aspirin-induced asthma: advances in pathogenesis, diagnosis and management. J Allergy Clin Immunol 2003;111:913–21.
8. Singh R, Gupta S, Dastidar S, et al. Cysteinyl leukotrienes and their receptors: molecular and functional characteristics. Pharmacology 2010;85:336–49.
9. Stevenson D, Szczeklik A. Clinical and pathologic perspectives on aspirin sensitivity and asthma. J Allergy Clin Immunol 2006;118:773–86.
10. Szczeklik A, Sladek K, Dworski R, et al. Bronchial aspirin challenge causes specific eicosanoid response in aspirin-sensitive asthmatics. Am J Respir Crit Care Med 1996;154:1608–14.

11. Christie P, Tagari P, Ford-Hutchinson A, et al. Urinary leukotrienes $E_4$ concentrations increase after aspirin challenge in aspirin-sensitive asthmatic subjects. Am Rev Respir Dis 1991;143:1025–9.
12. Smith C, Hawksworth R, Thien F, et al. Urinary leukotrienes $E_4$ in bronchial asthma. Eur Respir J 1992;5:693–9.
13. Sladek K, Dworski R, Soja J, et al. Eicosanoids in bronchoalveolar lavage fluid of aspirin intolerant patients with asthma after aspirin challenge. Am J Respir Crit Care Med 1994;149:940–6.
14. Antczak A, Montuschi P, Kharitonov S, et al. Increased exhaled cysteinyl-leukotrienes and 8-isoprostane in aspirin-induced asthma. Am J Respir Crit Care Med 2001;166:301–6.
15. Picado C, Ramis I, Rosello J, et al. Release of peptide leukotrienes into nasal secretions after local instillation of aspirin in aspirin-sensitive asthmatic patients. Am Rev Respir Dis 1992;145:65–9.
16. Nasser S, Pfister R, Christie P, et al. Inflammatory cell populations in bronchial biopsies from aspirin-sensitive asthmatic subjects. Am J Respir Crit Care Med 1996;153:90–6.
17. Cowburn A, Sladek K, Soja J, et al. Overexpression of leukotrienes $C_4$ synthase in bronchial biopsies from patients with aspirin-intolerant asthma. J Clin Invest 1998; 101(4):834–6.
18. Sousa A, Parikh A, Scadding M, et al. Leukotriene-receptor expression on nasal mucosal inflammatory cells in aspirin-sensitive rhinosinusitis. N Engl J Med 2002; 347:1493–9.
19. Daffern P, Muilenburg D, Jugli T, et al. Association of urinary leukotriene $E_4$ excretion during aspirin challenges with severity of respiratory responses. J Allergy Clin Immunol 1999;104:559–64.
20. Katial R, Strand M, Prasertsuntarasai T, et al. The effect of aspirin desensitization on novel biomarkers in aspirin-exacerbated respiratory diseases. J Allergy Clin Immunol 2010;126:738–44.
21. Hamilos D, Leung D, Wood R, et al. Evidence for distinct cytokine expression in allergic versus nonallergic chronic sinusitis. J Allergy Clin Immunol 1995;96: 537–44.
22. Riechelmann H, Deutschle T, Rozsasi A, et al. Nasal biomarker profiles in acute and chronic rhinosinusitis. Clin Exp Allergy 2005;35:1186–91.
23. Steinke J, Payne S, Borish L. Interleukin-4 in the generation of AERD phenotype: implications for molecular mechanisms driving therapeutic benefit of aspirin desensitization. J Allergy (Cairo) 2012;2012:182090.
24. Cianferoni A, Schroeder J, Kim J, et al. Selective inhibition of interleukin-4 gene expression in human T cells by aspirin. Blood 2001;97:1742–9.
25. Steinke J, Culp J, Kropf E, et al. Modulation by aspirin of nuclear phospho-signal transducer and activator of transcription 6 expression: possible role in therapeutic benefit associated with aspirin desensitization. J Allergy Clin Immunol 2009;124:724–30.
26. Vane J, Botting R. The mechanism of action of aspirin. Thromb Res 2003;110: 255–8.
27. Botting R. Vane's discovery of the mechanism of action of aspirin changed our understanding of its clinical pharmacology. Pharmacol Rep 2010;62:518–25.
28. Vane J. Inhibition of prostaglandin synthesis as a mechanism of action for aspirin-like drugs. Nat New Biol 1971;231(25):232–5.
29. Schafer D, Maune S. Pathogenic mechanisms and in vitro diagnosis of AERD. J Allergy (Cairo) 2012;2012:789232.

30. Botting R. Inhibitors of cyclooxygenases: mechanisms selectivity and uses. J Physiol Pharmacol 2006;57(Suppl 5):113–24.
31. Hall R, Mazer C. Antiplatelet drugs: a review of their pharmacology and management in the perioperative period. Anesth Analg 2011;112:292–318.
32. Lee T, Woszczek G, Farooque S. Leukotriene $E_4$: perspective on the forgotten mediator. J Allergy Clin Immunol 2009;124:417–21.
33. Arm J, O'Hickey S, Hawksworth R, et al. Asthmatic airways have disproportionate hyperresponsiveness to $LTE_4$, as compared with normal airways, but not to $LTC_4$, $LTD_4$, methacholine, and histamine. Am Rev Respir Dis 1990;142:1112–8.
34. Maekawa A, Kanaoka Y, Xing W, et al. Functional recognition of a distinct receptor preferential for leukotriene $E_4$ in mice lacking the cysteinyl leukotriene 1 and 2 receptors. Proc Natl Acad Sci U S A 2008;105:16695–700.
35. Paruchuri S, Tashimo H, Feng C, et al. Leukotriene $E_4$-induced pulmonary inflammation is mediated by the $P2Y_{12}$ receptor. J Exp Med 2009;206:2543–55.
36. Nasser S, Patel M, Bell G, et al. The effect of aspirin desensitization on urinary leukotriene $E_4$ concentrations in aspirin-sensitive asthma. Am J Respir Crit Care Med 1995;151:1326–30.
37. Arm J, O'Hickey S, Spur B, et al. Airway responsiveness to histamine and leukotriene E4 in subjects with aspirin-induced asthma. Am Rev Respir Dis 1989;140:148–53.
38. Juergens U, Christiansen M, Stevenson D, et al. Inhibition of monocyte leukotriene $B_4$ production after aspirin desensitization. J Allergy Clin Immunol 1995;96:148–56.
39. Perez-Novo C, Watelet J, Claeys C, et al. Prostaglandin, leukotriene, and lipoxin balance in chronic rhinosinusitis with and without nasal polyposis. J Allergy Clin Immunol 2005;115:1189–96.
40. Serhan C. Lipoxins and aspirin-triggered 15-epi-lipoxins are the first lipid mediators of endogenous anti-inflammation and resolution. Prostaglandins Leukot Essent Fatty Acids 2005;73:141–62.
41. Szczeklik A, Sanak M, Nizankowska-Mogilnicka E, et al. Aspirin intolerance and the cyclooxygenase leukotriene pathways. Curr Opin Pulm Med 2004;10:51–8.
42. Edenius C, Kumlin M, Bjork T, et al. Lipoxin formation in human nasal polyps and bronchial tissue. FEBS Lett 1990;272:25–8.
43. Sanak M, Levy B, Clish C, et al. Aspirin-tolerant asthmatics generate more lipoxins than aspirin-intolerant asthmatics. Eur Respir J 2000;16:44–9.
44. Claria J, Serhan CN. Aspirin triggers previously undescribed bioactive eicosanoids by human endothelial cell-leukocyte interactions. Proc Natl Acad Sci U S A 1995;92:9475–9.
45. Ohira T, Bannenberg G, Arita M, et al. A stable aspirin-triggered liopxin $A_4$ analog blocks phosphorylation of leukocyte-specific protein 1 in human neutrophils. J Immunol 2004;173:2091–8.
46. Ridker P, Cook N, Lee I, et al. A randomized trial of low-dose aspirin in the primary prevention of cardiovascular disease in women. N Engl J Med 2005;352:1293–304.
47. Figueroa D, Dreyer R, Defoe S, et al. Expression of the cysteinyl leukotriene 1 receptor in normal human lung and peripheral blood leukocytes. Am J Respir Crit Care Med 2001;163:226–33.
48. Picado C. Aspirin intolerance and nasal polyposis. Curr Allergy Asthma Rep 2002;2:488–93.
49. Kelly-Welch A, Hanson E, Keegan A. Interleuin-4 (IL-4) pathway. Sci STKE 2005;2005(293):cm9.

50. Hsieh F, Lam B, Penrose J, et al. T helper cell type 2 cytokines coordinately regulate immunoglobulin E-dependent cysteinyl leukotriene production by human cord blood-derived mast cells: profound induction of leukotriene C4 synthase expression by interleukin 4. J Exp Med 2001;193:123–33.

51. Early S, Barekzi E, Negri J, et al. Concordant modulation of cysteinyl leukotriene receptor expression by IL-4 and IFN-γ on peripheral immune cells. Am J Respir Cell Mol Biol 2007;36:715–20.

52. Kaplan M, Wurster A, Smiley S, et al. STAT6-dependent and -independent pathways for IL-4 production. J Immunol 1999;163:6536–40.

53. Cho W, Kim Y, Jeoung D, et al. Il-4 and Il-13 suppress prostaglandins production in human follicular dendritic cells by repressing COX-2 and mPGES-1 expression through JAK1 and STAT6. Mol Immunol 2011;48:966–72.

54. Cho W, Jeoung D, Kim Y, et al. STAT6 and JAK1 are essential for IL-4 mediated suppression of prostaglandin production in human follicular dendritic cells: opposing roles of phosphorylated and unphosphorylated STAT6. Int Immunopharmacol 2012;12:635–42.

55. Perez-G M, Melo M, Keegan A, et al. Aspirin and salicylates inhibit the IL-4 and IL-13 induced activation of STAT6. J Immunol 2002;168:1428–34.

56. Yamashita T, Tsuyi H, Maeda N, et al. Etiology of nasal polyps associated with aspirin-sensitive asthma. Rhinology 1989;8:15–24.

57. Kowalski ML, Grzegorczyk J, Wojciechowska B, et al. Intranasal challenge with aspirin induces cell influx and activation of eosinophils and mast cells in nasal secretions of ASA-sensitive patients. Clin Exp Allergy 1996;26:807–14.

58. Nasser S, Christie P, Pfister R, et al. Effect of endobronchial aspirin challenge on inflammatory cells in bronchial biopsy samples from aspirin-sensitive asthmatic subjects. Thorax 1996;51:64–70.

59. Bosso J, Schwartz L, Stevenson D. Tryptase and histamine release during aspirin-induced respiratory reactions. J Allergy Clin Immunol 1991;88:830–7.

60. Fischer A, Mitchell R, Lilly C, et al. Direct evidence for a role of the mast cell in the nasal response to aspirin in aspirin-sensitive asthma. J Allergy Clin Immunol 1994;94:1046–56.

61. Barr R, Kurth T, Stampfer M, et al. Aspirin and decreased adult-onset asthma: randomized comparisons from the physicians' health study. Am J Respir Crit Care Med 2007;175:120–5.

62. Kopp E, Ghosh S. Inhibition of NF-κβ by sodium salicylate and aspirin. Science 1994;265:956–9.

63. Yin M, Yamamoto Y, Gaynor R. The anti-inflammatory agents aspirin and salicylate inhibit the activity of Iκβ kinase-β. Nature 1998;369:77–80.

64. Schwenger P, Alpert D, Skolnik EY, et al. Activation of p38 mitogen-activated protein kinase by sodium salicylate leads to inhibition of tumor necrosis factor-induced Iκβα phosphorylation and degradation. Mol Cell Biol 1998;18: 78–84.

65. Aceves M, Duenas A, Gomez C, et al. A new pharmacological effect of salicylates: inhibition of NFAT-dependent transcription. J Immunol 2004;173:5721–9.

66. Dong A, Huang C, Brown R, et al. Inhibition of activator protein-1 activity and neoplastic transformation by aspirin. J Biol Chem 1997;272:9962–70.

67. Hawley S, Fullerton M, Ross F, et al. The ancient drug salicylate directly activates AMP-activated protein kinase. Science 2012;336:918–22.

68. Din F, Valanciute A, Houde V, et al. Aspirin inhibits mTOR signaling, activates AMP-activated protein kinase, and induces autophagy in colorectal cancer cells. Gastroenterology 2012;142:1504–15.

# NSAID Single-Drug–Induced Reactions

Katharine M. Woessner, MD[a],*, Mariana Castells, MD[b]

## KEYWORDS

- Nonsteroidal anti-inflammatory drugs (NSAIDs) • Adverse drug reactions (ADRs)
- Stevens-Johnson syndrome (SJS) • Toxic epidermal necrolysis (TEN)
- Drug rash with eosinophilia and systemic symptoms (DRESS)
- Acute generalized erythematous pustulosis (AGEP)

## KEY POINTS

- Nonsteroidal anti-inflammatory drugs (NSAIDs) are cyclooxygenase (COX) inhibitors with important analgesic, anti-inflammatory, antipyretic, and antithrombotic effects.
- NSAIDs have been implicated in a variety of drug-induced reactions that are proved as or suspected of being mediated through a host immune response.
- The types of single-drug–induced reactions are the confluence of 2 variables, namely the structure of the drug and the specific types of the immune responses.

## INTRODUCTION

NSAIDs are the most commonly prescribed class of drugs in the world and implicated in 20% to 25% of all adverse drug reactions (ADRs), second only to antibiotics.[1,2] ADRs are defined by the World Health Organization as any noxious, unintended, and undesired effect of a drug that occurs at doses used for prevention, diagnosis, or treatment. ADRs can be categorized into predictable (type A) and unpredictable (type B) reactions. Predictable reactions are usually dose dependent and related to the known pharmacologic actions of the drug and account for approximately 80% of all ADRs. They include overdose, side effects, secondary effects, and drug interactions. Unpredictable reactions are generally dose independent, are unrelated to pharmacologic actions of the drug, and occur only in susceptible subjects. These include drug intolerance (eg, tinnitus with aspirin at very low doses), drug allergy, drug

Disclosures: K.M.W: None; M.C: Consultant Merck, Sanofi: Adverse Drug Reactions Board Committee.
[a] Scripps Allergy and Immunology Fellowship Program, Division of Allergy and Immunology, Scripps Clinic, 3811 Valley Centre Drive, San Diego, CA 92130, USA; [b] Allergy and Clinical Immunology Training Program, Brigham and Women's Hospital, Harvard Medical School, 1 Jimmy Fund Way, Smith Building, Room 626D, Boston, MA 02115, USA
* Corresponding author.
E-mail address: Woessner.katharine@scrippshealth.org

idiosyncrasy, and pseudoallergic reactions. The focus of this article is on type B or unpredictable ADRs to NSAIDs.

NSAID-induced hypersensitivity reactions (HSRs) have a population prevalence of 0.3% to 2.5%.[1,3] These reactions can be manifested by asthma, rhinosinusitis, anaphylaxis, and/or urticaria and late-onset cutaneous and organ-specific reactions. Although there is no perfect classification system, the Gell and Coombs system of hypersensitivity can be used to classify the immunologically mediated reactions to NSAIDs. It includes immediate-type reactions mediated by drug-specific IgE antibodies (type I), cytotoxic reactions mediated by drug-specific IgG or IgM antibodies (type II), immune complex reactions (type III), and delayed-type HSRs mediated by cellular immune mechanisms (type IV).[4] Reactions to NSAIDs can be further classified based on the timing of the reaction, symptoms, and underlying mechanism (**Table 1**).

HSRs to all NSAIDS have been reported. The proprionic acid group of NSAIDs (naproxen, diclofenac, and ibuprofen) has a higher risk of anaphylactic reactions than other groups, which may reflect their longer presence in clinical use.[5,6] Ibuprofen is the most commonly prescribed NSAID in all age groups. Pyrazolones are the most likely NSAIDs to induce IgE-mediated HSRs/anaphylaxis.[7-9] The selective COX-2 inhibitors can also induce HSRs although the estimated incidence is low, at 0.008%.[10] Although the prevalence of delayed-type cutaneous reactions to NSAIDs is not known, severe reactions, such as erythema multiforme, toxic epidermal necrolyis (TEN), Stevens-Johnson syndrome (SJS), or drug reaction with eosinophilia and systemic symptoms (DRESS), have been reported.[11] The focus of this article is on single NSAID reactors. As many as 30% of patients with a history of an HSR to NSAIDs are estimated as single-drug reactors.[6]

Single-agent HSRs to aspirin can occur in some patients with cutaneous and systemic mastocytosis, inducing symptoms of mast cell activation, such as nasal congestion, shortness of breath with wheezing, and, in rare cases, hypotension and anaphylaxis. All patients with mastocytosis should undergo a diagnostic challenge with aspirin to assess tolerance to aspirin. Aspirin is used therapeutically in mastocytosis to block prostaglandin generation and, thereby, induce a dramatic reduction of flushing and central nervous system symptoms in these patients.[12]

## URTICARIA/ANGIOEDEMA/ANAPHYLAXIS

Selective NSAID acute HSRs have many features resembling type I hypersensitivity, although the identification of specific IgE antibody is usually not found.[13] In anecdotal cases, however, demonstration either of a positive skin test or specific IgE to albumin-bound aspirin has been found.[14,15] The participation of mast cells in these reactions has been demonstrated by finding products of mast cell activation, including elevated serum tryptase levels.[16] Any of the following clinical manifestations may be observed after oral, topical, or injected exposure to a single NSAID: urticaria, angioedema, laryngeal edema, generalized itching, rhinitis, bronchospasm, anaphylaxis, and even death. As discussed previously, reactions to a single NSAID are seen more often in patients treated with NSAIDs in the pyrazolone class.[7,17] Reports for most of the other NSAIDs, however, including acetaminophen, aspirin, celecoxib, fenoprofen, indomethacin, ketorolac, meclofenamate, naproxen, piroxicam, tolmetin, sulindac, and zomepirac, are available.[18] In single-drug reactions to acetaminophen, generalized urticaria and angioedema are the most common symptoms, although anaphylactic shock has been described.[19,20]

A critical feature of single-drug HSRs is tolerance of other chemically unrelated NSAIDs, which strongly argues against a role of COX inhibition in the pathophysiology

**Table 1**
Classification of hypersensitivity reactions to NSAIDs

| Timing of Reaction | Clinical Features | Type of Reaction | Underlying Disease | Possible Mechanism |
|---|---|---|---|---|
| Acute (within minutes to hours after exposure) | Rhinitis/asthma | Cross reactive | Asthma, sinusitis, nasal polyps | COX-1 Inhibition |
| | Urticaria/angioedema | Cross reactive | Chronic urticaria | COX-1 inhibition |
| | Urticaria/angioedema | Cross reactive | No underlying chronic disease | ? COX-1 inhibition |
| | Urticaria/angioedema/anaphylaxis | Single-drug induced | Atopy | Type 1 hypersensitivity |
| Delayed (>24 h after exposure) | Fixed drug eruptions, drug exanthems, SJS toxic epidermolysis, pneumonitis, aseptic meningitis, contact and photoallergic dermatitis | Single-drug induced (or in same chemical class) | No underlying disease | T-cell–mediated type IV type hypersensitivity, cytotoxic T cells, natural killer cells, other |

*Modified from* Goodwin SD, Glenny RW. Nonsteroidal anti-inflammatory drug-associated pulmonary infiltrates with eosinophilia. Review of the literature and Food and Drug Administration Adverse Drug Reaction reports. Arch Intern Med 1992;152:1521-4.

of these reactions. Positive skin tests to a culprit drug or serum IgE may be found in a large number of pyrazolone reactors.[14] Unfortunately, this is rarely the case for other single NSAID reactors. A recent study of 41 subjects with history of anaphylaxis to diclofenac failed to identify specific IgE to the drug or its phase 1 metabolites.[21] It is of critical importance to identify patients who are the single NSAID reactor so as to not indiscriminately eliminate all future use of innocent NSAIDs.

Diagnosing single NSAID reactors is challenging. With the exception of pyrazolones, there are no standardized skin tests of in vitro assays available to diagnose NSAID hypersensitivity. Furthermore, relying solely on patient history is an unreliable source of information. This was confirmed in a recent study by Viola and colleagues[22] that assessed NSAID hypersensitivity in 275 patients by provocation tests in which they found that 77.8% of their subjects with a historical reaction to an NSAID tolerated that NSAID in an oral challenge whereas only 22.2% reacted (the study excluded patients with aspirin exacerbated respiratory disease). In the absence of a reliable in vitro test, the accurate diagnosis of NSAID hypersensitivity depends on a careful history and oral drug challenge/provocation testing. In patients with a history of severe reactions (anaphylactic shock), an oral provocation test with the culprit drug should almost never be performed because the risk versus benefit favors selecting another NSAID. In those individuals, oral challenge with unrelated NSAIDs and aspirin should be undertaken to rule out cross-reactive hypersensitivity and confirm the safety of an alternative NSAID.

Once the diagnosis of a single-drug reaction is confirmed, the avoidance of that particular drug and other chemically similar NSAIDs should be advised. An exception is aspirin due to its unique antiplatelet effects. Aspirin has been reported in the literature as a historical cause of anaphylaxis in patients seen in emergency rooms.[23] There are 2 reports of positive skin tests to lysyl aspirin in patients with aspirin-induced urticaria.[15,24] These observations suggest that aspirin-induced anaphylaxis is a possibility. Yet, despite an extensive literature search and careful review, peer consultation throughout multiple medical systems, and an exhaustive review of the cases of aspirin reactions in the Scripps medical system, the authors have been unable to find even one convincing case of an anaphylactic reaction to aspirin (see the article by Woessner and Simon elsewhere in this issue for further details). A summary of the approach to management of single NSAIDs type I HSRs is available in **Box 1**.

## DELAYED REACTIONS TO NSAIDS

The group of delayed NSAID-specific reactions includes exanthems, pustular and bullous reactions, and organ-specific reactions (**Box 2**). T lymphocytes play a key role in the pathogenesis with drug specificity the hallmark of these reactions.

### Drug-Induced Maculopapular Exanthema

Maculopapular exanthem is the most common type of drug-induced cutaneous reaction. The term describes a usually faint and mild cutaneous eruption that exhibits the combined characteristics of macules (discolored areas of skin that are not elevated above the surface) and papules (small, solid, usually inflammatory elevations of the skin that do not contain pus). The rash is often referred to as morbilliform (in resembling the dusky red eruption of measles). These cutaneous reactions often begin on the trunk and pressure-bearing areas and then progress, becoming confluent and covering large areas of the body.[25] Maculopapular eruptions often have a characteristic structure, with widespread lesions on the upper torso or head and neck. They often have a symmetric pattern of pinpoint pink to red papules that can coalesce,

---

**Box 1**

**Diagnosis and management of type I hypersensitivity reactions to NSAIDs**

*Diagnosis*

1. Symptoms of type I HSRs to NSAIDs: urticaria, angioedema, anaphylaxis

2. Check serum tryptase at time of reaction to assess mast cell activation

3. Challenge with culprit drug if historical reaction urticaria or angioedema only

4. If history of anaphylaxis: avoid challenge of culprit drug

   a. Exception: aspirin[a]

5. Determine if due to COX inhibition (cross-reactivity vs single NSAID)

   a. Challenge with acetylsalicylic acid (aspirin) or other nonculprit NSAID

      i. Positive challenge indicative of cross-reacting and not single NSAID HSRs

      ii. Negative challenge: no cross-reactivity, confirms single NSAID HSRs

*Recommendations for confirmed single NSAID HSRs*

1. Avoid culprit drug

2. Safe to use all other NSAIDs (with negative cross-reactivity challenge)

3. If aspirin needed for antiplatelet effects, may challenge/desensitize[a]

4. Medical alert bracelet with accurate information regarding NSAIDs avoidance

5. Injectable epinephrine for patients with history of anaphylaxis

[a] See article by Woessner and Simon in this issue.

---

yielding a rough or coarse texture. Patients may also experience moderate to severe pruritus and fever.[25] Most drug-induced maculopapular exanthems are mild, appearing 8 to 10 days after initiation of drug therapy (but can be earlier or later) and fade within a similar period after medication withdrawal.

---

**Box 2**

**Selective delayed reactions to NSAIDs (T-cell mediated)**

1. Maculopapular exanthema

2. Fixed drug eruptions

3. Acute generalized exanthematous pustulosis (AGEP)

4. Severe bullous cutaneous reactions

   a. SJS

   b. TEN

5. DRESS

6. Organ-specific reactions

   a. Hepatitis

   b. Nephritis

   c. Hypersensitivity pneumonitis

   d. Aseptic meningitis

---

These mild cutaneous reactions, however, also rarely represent the early manifestation of rare, severe drug-induced cutaneous reactions, such as SJS and TEN, which result in epidermal detachment and have high rates of morbidity and mortality.[26] Therefore, withdrawal of the offending treatment is imperative in patients with maculopapular exanthems.[26]

### Fixed Drug Eruptions

The term, *fixed drug eruption*, describes the development of 1 or more annular or oval erythematous patches as a result of systemic exposure to a drug; these reactions normally resolve with hyperpigmentation and may recur at the same site with re-exposure to the drug. Repeated exposure to the offending drug may cause new lesions to develop in addition to lighting up the older hyperpigmented lesions. NSAIDs are among the most common causes of fixed drug eruptions.[27,28]

### Acute Generalized Exanthematous Pustulosis

AGEP is characterized by the rapid appearance of many pustules, which are sterile and located subcorneally in the epidermis; the patients have fever, leukocytosis, and sometimes eosinophilia. AGEP resolves quickly with withdrawal of the drug. It has been reported with several NSAIDs, including nimsulide, ibuprofen, and celecoxib.[29–31]

### Severe Bullous Cutaneous Reactions: SJS and TEN

SJS and TEN represent a spectrum, with extent of detachment of skin (percentage of total body surface) determining the nomenclature: SJS (<10%), SJS/TEN overlap (10%–30%), and TEN (>30%).[11] This severe cutaneous reaction is extremely rare, potentially fatal, and frequently associated with certain newly prescribed drugs. Symptoms can occur 1 to 8 weeks after administration of incriminated drugs.[11] For some patients, an initial diagnosis of SJS may be replaced with a diagnosis of extensive TEN if there is disease progression. The clinical findings include a painful generalized cutaneous eruption progressing in days to blisters, which are quickly followed by detachment of large sheets of epidermis. Additionally, mucosal inflammation (conjunctivae, mouth, esophagus, vaginal tract, and so forth) occurs in all cases. Systemic symptoms of fever and fatigue, hepatitis and nephritis also occur, particularly at the more severe end of the above spectrum.

Early withdrawal of the offending agent is essential in obtaining a favorable outcome: morbidity and mortality rates may increase in instances in which withdrawal is delayed.[32] An association between onset of SJS/TEN and a single, newly prescribed drug has been well established.[33] Because physician-ordered rechallenge with a suspect drug is never indicated, however, the precise identification of a specific drug reaction is frequently in doubt. Drug prescribing patterns and, therefore, association patterns are different. For antibiotics, such as sulfonamides, penicillins, cephalosporins, and quinolones, and some NSAIDs (acetaminophen, ibuprofen, and naproxen), these drugs are usually prescribed and taken for short periods of time. Therefore, the onset of the initial rash usually begins near the end or shortly after the conclusion of treatment.[33] For other drugs, such as allopurinol, carbamazepine, phenytoin, phenobarbital, valproic acid, and NSAIDS, long-term prescribing patterns are more common. Oxicams are the NSAIDs most frequently implicated in this uncommon type of reaction. Other reported NSAIDs include phenylbutazone and selective COX-2 inhibitors.[10,11,33] The highest risk for these rare reactions is in the time frame of 1 to 8 weeks, with a mean of approximately 2 weeks, after initiating treatment.[1,3] Furthermore, there is a sharp drop-off in incidence of SJS/TEN after a drug has been taken daily for longer than 2 months.

Determining the culprit drug is most difficult in patients on long-term treatment with polypharmacy. Patients hospitalized with SJS/TEN, when the admitting drugs list includes 2 or more continuously ingested drugs, are diagnostically challenging. Standard practice is to discontinue all drugs, while acknowledging that only 1, and maybe none, of the drugs on the list caused SJS/TEN in the first place. This situation is further complicated by SJS/TEN reactions also being able to be activated by certain infections, in particular but not limited to mycoplasma pneumoniae and herpes simplex virus. A recent study in Korea of all patients admitted to the Kyungpook National University Hospital from 2001 to 2011 with a diagnosis of SJS or TEN reported that in 82 patients (71 SJS and 11 TEN), drug associations were identified in 43 patients (53.4%) whereas in 39/82 (47.5%), no drug association could be found.[34] In some of these patients, obvious mycoplasma or viral infections preceded the onset of SJS/TEN, but in others, the patients consumed no drug and no other cause was apparent (idiopathic).

Given that reintroduction of a suspect drug might induce a severe if not fatal reaction and that a reliable in vitro test has not been developed, many innocent bystander drugs are now listed in the *Physicians' Desk Reference* or computer data sources as causing SJS/TEN. With millions of people throughout the world taking aspirin (81 or 325 mg once a day) for cardiovascular protection, the chances of a misattribution of aspirin as a cause of SJS/TEN are significant. Despite aspirin's frequent listing as one of the drugs in the suspect polypharmacy, it is unlikely that aspirin has ever been a causative drugs for inducing SJS/TEN.[35]

Patients with extensive severe skin reactions should also be treated as burn patients, with use of fluid resuscitation, infection control measures, and nutritional support in a hospital burn unit setting.[36] The use of corticosteroids is controversial.[26,37,38] If treatment is delayed, it is possible that TEN could supervene, in which case systemic corticosteroids are contraindicated.[26,39] The effects of intravenous immunoglobulin (IVIG) have also been investigated for the treatment of TEN, with some studies showing an improved outcome.[40–43] Other studies using high-dose IVIG have failed to show an improved outcome.[44,45] The proposed mechanism of action of IVIG is inhibition of FAS-FAS ligand–associated apoptosis of keratinocytes seen in TEN.[46] There are some reports that use of anti–tumor necrosis factor α may be beneficial.[47,48]

After surviving SJS/TEN, standard practice is to educate patients to avoid suspect drugs for the rest of a patient's life. In cases of polypharmacy, accurately determining the clinically relevant culprit drug may be impossible. If any of these long-term drugs is essential for a patient's survival and difficult or even impossible to replace, obtaining informed consent and reintroduction is within the standard of care. For NSAIDs, however, this only applies when aspirin is one of the discontinued drugs and other suspect drugs or infections are available to explain the reaction. Due to the unique antiplatelet effects of aspirin, other NSAIDs are not interchangeable. Fortunately, there is no convincing evidence that aspirin has ever caused SJS/TEN.[35] For all other implicated NSAIDs, substitution of another NSAID from a different class is appropriate and is the standard of care.

## Drug Rash with Eosinophilia and Systemic Symptoms

Drug-induced hypersensitivity syndrome, or DRESS syndrome, is a serious acute drug reaction that is characterized by fever, cutaneous eruption, and involvement of several internal organs in the form of enlarged lymph nodes, hepatitis, renal impairment, pneumonitis, carditis, and hematologic abnormalities (mainly hypereosinophilia and atypical lymphocytosis).[26,49] DRESS can start 2 to 8 weeks after initiating drug therapy and symptoms may even worsen when the suspect drug is discontinued. DRESS has been reported in patients taking ibuprofen or phenylbutazone, and, more recently, celecoxib.[50,51] There is only 1 case report of DRESS associated with use of aspirin in a child treated for Kawasaki disease confirmed by skin patch testing.[52] This is unusual because of the nonassociation of aspirin in any other CD8+ T-lymphocyte–mediated delayed reactions and was not confirmed with rechallenge with aspirin.

DRESS is an atypical drug allergic reaction in which the symptoms can be progressive despite stopping the culprit drug.[53] Treatment includes stopping the offending drug and initiating use of corticosteroids. Limited data exist with regard to use of other agents, such as IVIG and immunomodulatory agents.[54]

### Hypersensitivity Pneumonitis

Development of a hypersensitivity pneumonitis has been associated with sulindac, ibuprofen, and naproxen.[55–57] Presenting features include fever, cough, dyspnea, and pulmonary infiltrates. Treatment involves stopping the culprit drug and, in some cases, initiation of treatment with systemic corticosteroids. To date, aspirin has not been implicated as a culprit drug for this type of reaction.

### Aseptic Meningitis

This type of drug hypersensitivity, aseptic meningitis, is more frequently observed in patients with a history of autoimmune diseases, in particular, systemic lupus erythematosus.[58–60] Diagnosis is by exclusion of an infectious agent and other noninfectious causes and by demonstrating a convincing temporal relationship between ingestion of a specific drug and the onset of symptoms.[58,59] Treatment is stopping the culprit drug. Several NSAIDs, including ibuprofen (most commonly) and sulindac, naproxen, tolmetin, diclofenac, ketoprofen, piroxicam, indomethacin, rofecoxib, and celecoxib, have been associated with aseptic meningitis.[61] Aspirin has not been reported with this syndrome. This is a drug-specific phenomenon in that these patients can tolerate other unrelated NSAIDs.[61,62]

### Contact and Photoallergic Dermatitis

Allergic contact dermatitis can occur with many NSAIDS. It appears as an itchy rash with erythematous papules, edema, and vesicles at sites of contact. Commonly involved NSAIDs include diclofenac, indomethacin, flurbiprofen, ibuprofen, ketoprofen, and tiaprofenic acid.[63,64] Photoallergic dermatitis is a T-cell–dependent reaction in which the culprit allergen needs to be activated by UV light to generate the reaction. The most common NSAIDs involved in this reaction are proprionic acid derivatives and oxicams.[65] Topical ketoprofen can be associated with both allergic contact dermatitis and photoallergic dermatitis.[66] Patients who develop contact dermatitis to a specific NSAID can experience severe cutaneous reactions if they take the drug orally, a syndrome known as systemic contact dermatitis. The skin reaction may occur within a few hours to days after systemic exposure to the drug and can present with a variable picture of symmetric widespread maculopapular rash, flare-up of previous dermatitis, flexural dermatitis, baboon syndrome, vasculitis-like lesion, erythema multiforme, or intractable eczema.[67,68] Systemic symptoms, such as headache, fever, malaise, arthralgia, vomiting, and diarrhea, may occur.[67] This has been described in association with diclofenac and valdecoxib.[69,70]

## DIAGNOSIS AND MANAGEMENT OF DELAYED REACTIONS TO NSAIDS

The diagnosis of delayed reactions to NSAIDs is dependent on taking a careful history and assessing the clinical picture. Useful testing modalities may include patch testing for suspected T-cell–mediated reactions. The patches are placed with petrolatum and readings are conducted at 24 to 48 hours.[71] There are case reports of patch testing as useful in fixed drug eruptions, DRESS, and AGEP.[71] For fixed drug eruptions, the drug must be applied to the site where the original reaction occurred.[72] For suspected photoallergic reactions, photo patch testing is indicated.[73]

The gold standard for diagnosis of drug hypersensitivity is oral provocation test with the suspect drug. Use of the suspect drug is contraindicated in patients with severe generalized reactions, such as AGEP, DRESS, and SJS/TEN.[74] An exception would be for aspirin that has been consumed for longer than 2 months without reactions in patients with other obvious suspect drugs or suspect infections (such as mycoplasma in SJS/TEN). In that situation, informed consent and challenge with aspirin are within the standard of care.

### Cardiac Toxicity and COX-2 Inhibitors

Concern over the safety of selective COX-2 inhibitors was raised with the data from the Vioxx Gastrointestinal Outcomes Research trial, which found a 5-fold increase in the incidence of myocardial infarction and stroke among patients taking rofecoxib compared with naproxen.[75] It was initially hypothesized that the increase was due to the cardioprotective effects of naproxen as opposed to cardiotoxic effects of rofecoxib. Subsequent meta-analysis of naproxen studies has failed to show a significant cardioprotective effect of naproxen, making this an unlikely explanation of the outcomes.[76,77] Subsequent trials with rofecoxib, including the Adenomatous Polyp Prevention on Vioxx trial, also demonstrated an unacceptable increase in cardiovascular events.[78]

Regarding celecoxib, there has been a single trial that demonstrated an increased cardiovascular risk at high doses (400 mg twice a day) but a consistent adverse effect has not been observed.[79–82] In 2005, the Food and Drug Administration decided that celecoxib should remain on the market. Graham and colleagues,[77] of the Food and Drug Administration, analyzed cardiovascular events in more than 1 million subjects, 26,748 of whom took rofecoxib and 40,405 of whom took celecoxib, and found that rofecoxib tripled the risk of cardiovascular events and that celecoxib did not significantly alter the cardiovascular risk. It has been proposed that the deleterious cardiovascular effects of rofecoxib are due to cardiotoxicity. Specifically, rofecoxib metabolites form a highly reactive maleic anhydride derivative that causes oxidative damage in various biologic targets, including human low-density lipoprotein and arachidonic acid, to form atherogenic aldehydes and isoprostanes, which was not seen with celecoxib.[83]

## REFERENCES

1. Gomes ER, Demoly P. Epidemiology of hypersensitivity drug reactions. Curr Opin Allergy Clin Immunol 2005;5:309–16.
2. Nettis E, Colanardi MC, Ferrannini A, et al. Update on sensitivity to nonsteroidal antiinflammatory drugs. Curr Drug Targets Immune Endocr Metabol Disord 2001;1:233–40.
3. Settipane RA, Constantine HP, Settipane GA. Aspirin intolerance and recurrent urticaria in normal adults and children. Epidemiology and review. Allergy 1980; 35:149–54.
4. Khan DA, Solensky R. Drug allergy. J Allergy Clin Immunol 2010;125:S126–37.

5. van Puijenbroek EP, Egberts AC, Meyboom RH, et al. Different risks for NSAID-induced anaphylaxis. Ann Pharmacother 2002;36:24–9.
6. Quiralte J, Blanco C, Delgado J, et al. Challenge-based clinical patterns of 223 Spanish patients with nonsteroidal anti-inflammatory-drug-induced-reactions. J Investig Allergol Clin Immunol 2007;17:182–8.
7. Van der Klauw MM, Wilson JH, Stricker BH. Drug-associated anaphylaxis: 20 years of reporting in The Netherlands (1974-1994) and review of the literature. Clin Exp Allergy 1996;26:1355–63.
8. Szczeklik A. Analgesics, allergy and asthma. Drugs 1986;32(Suppl 4):148–63.
9. Gomez E, Blanca-Lopez N, Torres MJ, et al. Immunoglobulin E-mediated immediate allergic reactions to dipyrone: value of basophil activation test in the identification of patients. Clin Exp Allergy 2009;39:1217–24.
10. Layton D, Marshall V, Boshier A, et al. Serious skin reactions and selective COX-2 inhibitors: a case series from prescription-event monitoring in England. Drug Saf 2006;29:687–96.
11. Mockenhaupt M, Kelly JP, Kaufman D, et al. The risk of Stevens-Johnson syndrome and toxic epidermal necrolysis associated with nonsteroidal antiinflammatory drugs: a multinational perspective. J Rheumatol 2003;30:2234–40.
12. Escribano L, Akin C, Castells M, et al. Mastocytosis: current concepts in diagnosis and treatment. Ann Hematol 2002;81:677–90.
13. Stevenson DD. Aspirin and NSAID sensitivity. Immunol Allergy Clin North Am 2004;24:491–505.
14. Czerniawska-Mysik G, Szczeklik A. Idiosyncrasy to pyrazolone drugs. Allergy 1981;36:381–4.
15. Blanca M, Perez E, Garcia JJ, et al. Angioedema and IgE antibodies to aspirin: a case report. Ann Allergy 1989;62:295–8.
16. Schwartz LB, Metcalfe DD, Miller JS, et al. Tryptase levels as an indicator of mast-cell activation in systemic anaphylaxis and mastocytosis. N Engl J Med 1987;316:1622–6.
17. Asero R. Oral aspirin challenges in patients with a history of intolerance to single non-steroidal anti-inflammatory drugs. Clin Exp Allergy 2005;35:713–6.
18. Sanchez-Borges M. NSAID hypersensitivity (respiratory, cutaneous, and generalized anaphylactic symptoms). Med Clin North Am 2010;94:853–64.
19. de Paramo BJ, Gancedo SQ, Cuevas M, et al. Paracetamol (acetaminophen) hypersensitivity. Ann Allergy Asthma Immunol 2000;85:508–11.
20. Liao CM, Chen WC, Lin CY. Study of an anaphylactoid reaction to acetaminophen. Acta Paediatr Taiwan 2002;43:147–52.
21. Harrer A, Lang R, Grims R, et al. Diclofenac hypersensitivity: antibody responses to the parent drug and relevant metabolites. PLoS One 2010;5:e13707.
22. Viola M, Rumi G, Valluzzi RL, et al. Assessing potential determinants of positive provocation tests in subjects with NSAID hypersensitivity. Clin Exp Allergy 2011;41:96–103.
23. Kemp SF, Lockey RF, Wolf BL, et al. Anaphylaxis. A review of 266 cases. Arch Intern Med 1995;155:1749–54.
24. Phills JA, Perelmutter L. IgE mediated and non-IgE mediated allergic-type reactions to aspirin. Acta Allergol 1974;29:474–90.
25. Svensson CK, Cowen EW, Gaspari AA. Cutaneous drug reactions. Pharmacol Rev 2001;53:357–79.
26. Roujeau JC, Stern RS. Severe adverse cutaneous reactions to drugs. N Engl J Med 1994;331:1272–85.
27. Savin JA. Current causes of fixed drug eruption in the UK. Br J Dermatol 2001; 145:667–8.

28. Mahboob A, Haroon TS. Drugs causing fixed eruptions: a study of 450 cases. Int J Dermatol 1998;37:833–8.
29. Yesudian PD, Penny M, Azurdia RM, et al. Ibuprofen-induced acute generalized exanthematous pustulosis. Int J Dermatol 2004;43:208–10.
30. Teixeira M, Silva E, Selores M. Acute generalized exanthematous pustulosis induced by nimesulide. Dermatol Online J 2006;12:20.
31. Pakdeethai J, Ho SA, Aw D, et al. Acute generalized exanthematous pustulosis-like, folliculitic drug reaction pattern caused by celecoxib. Dermatol Ther 2011; 24:505–7.
32. Ghislain PD, De Beir A, Creusy C, et al. Keratosis lichenoides chronica: report of a new case, with success of PUVA therapy. Dermatol Online J 2001;7:4.
33. Mockenhaupt M, Viboud C, Dunant A, et al. Stevens-Johnson syndrome and toxic epidermal necrolysis: assessment of medication risks with emphasis on recently marketed drugs. The EuroSCAR-study. J Invest Dermatol 2008;128:35–44.
34. Kim HI, Kim SW, Park GY, et al. Causes and treatment outcomes of Stevens-Johnson syndrome and toxic epidermal necrolysis in 82 adult patients. Korean J Intern Med 2012;27:203–10.
35. Kaufman DW, Kelly JP. Acetylsalicylic acid and other salicylates in relation to Stevens-Johnson syndrome and toxic epidermal necrolysis. Br J Clin Pharmacol 2001;51:174–6.
36. Kelemen JJ 3rd, Cioffi WG, McManus WF, et al. Burn center care for patients with toxic epidermal necrolysis. J Am Coll Surg 1995;180:273–8.
37. Cheriyan S, Patterson R, Greenberger PA, et al. The outcome of Stevens-Johnson syndrome treated with corticosteroids. Allergy Proc 1995;16:151–5.
38. Fine JD. Management of acquired bullous skin diseases. N Engl J Med 1995;333: 1475–84.
39. Becker DS. Toxic epidermal necrolysis. Lancet 1998;351:1417–20.
40. Viard I, Wehrli P, Bullani R, et al. Inhibition of toxic epidermal necrolysis by blockade of CD95 with human intravenous immunoglobulin. Science 1998;282:490–3.
41. Prins C, Kerdel FA, Padilla RS, et al. Treatment of toxic epidermal necrolysis with high-dose intravenous immunoglobulins: multicenter retrospective analysis of 48 consecutive cases. Arch Dermatol 2003;139:26–32.
42. Trent JT, Kerdel FA. Intravenous immunoglobulin for the treatment of toxic epidermal necrolysis. Arch Dermatol 2003;139:1081.
43. Trent JT, Kirsner RS, Romanelli P, et al. Analysis of intravenous immunoglobulin for the treatment of toxic epidermal necrolysis using SCORTEN: the University of Miami experience. Arch Dermatol 2003;139:39–43.
44. Bachot N, Revuz J, Roujeau JC. Intravenous immunoglobulin treatment for Stevens-Johnson syndrome and toxic epidermal necrolysis: a prospective non-comparative study showing no benefit on mortality or progression. Arch Dermatol 2003;139:33–6.
45. Shortt R, Gomez M, Mittman N, et al. Intravenous immunoglobulin does not improve outcome in toxic epidermal necrolysis. J Burn Care Rehabil 2004;25: 246–55.
46. Paul C, Wolkenstein P, Adle H, et al. Apoptosis as a mechanism of keratinocyte death in toxic epidermal necrolysis. Br J Dermatol 1996;134:710–4.
47. Hunger RE, Hunziker T, Buettiker U, et al. Rapid resolution of toxic epidermal necrolysis with anti-TNF-alpha treatment. J Allergy Clin Immunol 2005;116:923–4.
48. Fischer M, Fiedler E, Marsch WC, et al. Antitumour necrosis factor-alpha antibodies (infliximab) in the treatment of a patient with toxic epidermal necrolysis. Br J Dermatol 2002;146:707–9.

49. Bocquet H, Bagot M, Roujeau JC. Drug-induced pseudolymphoma and drug hypersensitivity syndrome (Drug Rash with Eosinophilia and Systemic Symptoms: DRESS). Semin Cutan Med Surg 1996;15:250–7.
50. Um SJ, Lee SK, Kim YH, et al. Clinical features of drug-induced hypersensitivity syndrome in 38 patients. J Investig Allergol Clin Immunol 2010;20:556–62.
51. Lee JH, Park HK, Heo J, et al. Drug Rash with Eosinophilia and Systemic Symptoms (DRESS) syndrome induced by celecoxib and anti-tuberculosis drugs. J Korean Med Sci 2008;23:521–5.
52. Kawakami T, Fujita A, Takeuchi S, et al. Drug-induced hypersensitivity syndrome: drug reaction with eosinophilia and systemic symptoms (DRESS) syndrome induced by aspirin treatment of Kawasaki disease. J Am Acad Dermatol 2009; 60:146–9.
53. Joint Task Force on Practice Parameters, American Academy of Allergy, Asthma and Immunology, American College of Allergy, Asthma and Immunology, et al. Drug allergy: an updated practice parameter. Ann Allergy Asthma Immunol 2010;105:259–73.
54. Fields KS, Petersen MJ, Chiao E, et al. Case reports: treatment of nevirapine-associated dress syndrome with intravenous immune globulin (IVIG). J Drugs Dermatol 2005;4:510–3.
55. Allen JN. Drug-induced eosinophilic lung disease. Clin Chest Med 2004;25: 77–88.
56. Weber JC, Essigman WK. Pulmonary alveolitis and NSAIDs—fact or fiction? Br J Rheumatol 1986;25:5–6.
57. Goodwin SD, Glenny RW. Nonsteroidal anti-inflammatory drug-associated pulmonary infiltrates with eosinophilia. Review of the literature and Food and Drug Administration Adverse Drug Reaction reports. Arch Intern Med 1992;152: 1521–4.
58. Jolles S, Sewell WA, Leighton C. Drug-induced aseptic meningitis: diagnosis and management. Drug Saf 2000;22:215–26.
59. Moris G, Garcia-Monco JC. The challenge of drug-induced aseptic meningitis. Arch Intern Med 1999;159:1185–94.
60. Moreno-Ancillo A, Gil-Adrados AC, Jurado-Palomo J. Ibuprofen-induced aseptic meningoencephalitis confirmed by drug challenge. J Investig Allergol Clin Immunol 2011;21:484–7.
61. Ashwath ML, Katner HP. Recurrent aseptic meningitis due to different non-steroidal anti-inflammatory drugs including rofecoxib. Postgrad Med J 2003;79: 295–6.
62. Ballas ZK, Donta ST. Sulindac-induced aseptic meningitis. Arch Intern Med 1982; 142:165–6.
63. Kowalski ML, Makowska JS, Blanca M, et al. Hypersensitivity to nonsteroidal anti-inflammatory drugs (NSAIDs) - classification diagnosis and management: review of the EAACI/ENDA(#) and GA2LEN/HANNA*. Allergy 2011;66:818–29.
64. Pigatto PD, Mozzanica N, Bigardi AS, et al. Topical NSAID allergic contact dermatitis. Italian experience. Contact Derm 1993;29:39–41.
65. Gould JW, Mercurio MG, Elmets CA. Cutaneous photosensitivity diseases induced by exogenous agents. J Am Acad Dermatol 1995;33:551–73.
66. Bagheri H, Lhiaubet V, Montastruc JL, et al. Photosensitivity to ketoprofen: mechanisms and pharmacoepidemiological data. Drug Saf 2000;22:339–49.
67. Thyssen JP, Maibach HI. Drug-elicited systemic allergic (contact) dermatitis—update and possible pathomechanisms. Contact Derm 2008;59:195–202.

68. Posadas SJ, Pichler WJ. Delayed drug hypersensitivity reactions—new concepts. Clin Exp Allergy 2007;37:989–99.
69. Lakshmi C, Srinivas CR. Systemic (allergic) contact dermatitis to diclofenac. Indian J Dermatol Venereol Leprol 2011;77:536–40.
70. Jaeger C, Jappe U. Valdecoxib-induced systemic contact dermatitis confirmed by positive patch test. Contact Derm 2005;52:47–8.
71. Barbaud A. Skin testing in delayed reactions to drugs. Immunol Allergy Clin North Am 2009;29:517–35.
72. Shiohara T. Fixed drug eruption: pathogenesis and diagnostic tests. Curr Opin Allergy Clin Immunol 2009;9:316–21.
73. Hasan T, Jansen CT. Photopatch test reactivity: effect of photoallergen concentration and UVA dosaging. Contact Derm 1996;34:383–6.
74. Aberer W, Bircher A, Romano A, et al. Drug provocation testing in the diagnosis of drug hypersensitivity reactions: general considerations. Allergy 2003;58:854–63.
75. Bombardier C, Laine L, Reicin A, et al. Comparison of upper gastrointestinal toxicity of rofecoxib and naproxen in patients with rheumatoid arthritis. VIGOR Study Group. N Engl J Med 2000;343:1520–8.
76. Juni P, Nartey L, Reichenbach S, et al. Risk of cardiovascular events and rofecoxib: cumulative meta-analysis. Lancet 2004;364:2021–9.
77. Graham DJ, Campen D, Hui R, et al. Risk of acute myocardial infarction and sudden cardiac death in patients treated with cyclo-oxygenase 2 selective and non-selective non-steroidal anti-inflammatory drugs: nested case-control study. Lancet 2005;365:475–81.
78. Bresalier RS, Sandler RS, Quan H, et al. Cardiovascular events associated with rofecoxib in a colorectal adenoma chemoprevention trial. N Engl J Med 2005; 352:1092–102.
79. Solomon SD, McMurray JJ, Pfeffer MA, et al. Cardiovascular risk associated with celecoxib in a clinical trial for colorectal adenoma prevention. N Engl J Med 2005; 352:1071–80.
80. Ray WA, Stein CM, Daugherty JR, et al. COX-2 selective non-steroidal anti-inflammatory drugs and risk of serious coronary heart disease. Lancet 2002;360: 1071–3.
81. Solomon DH, Schneeweiss S, Glynn RJ, et al. Relationship between selective cyclooxygenase-2 inhibitors and acute myocardial infarction in older adults. Circulation 2004;109:2068–73.
82. Mamdani M, Juurlink DN, Lee DS, et al. Cyclo-oxygenase-2 inhibitors versus non-selective non-steroidal anti-inflammatory drugs and congestive heart failure outcomes in elderly patients: a population-based cohort study. Lancet 2004; 363:1751–6.
83. Mason RP, Walter MF, Day CA, et al. A biological rationale for the cardiotoxic effects of rofecoxib: comparative analysis with other COX-2 selective agents and NSAids. Subcell Biochem 2007;42:175–90.

# Aspirin-Exacerbated Cutaneous Disease

Mario Sánchez-Borges, MD*, Fernan Caballero-Fonseca, MD,
Arnaldo Capriles-Hulett, MD

## KEYWORDS

- Aspirin • Angioedema • Chronic urticaria • Cyclooxygenases • Leukotrienes
- NSAIDs

## KEY POINTS

- About one-third of patients with chronic urticaria experience exacerbation of cutaneous symptoms when they take aspirin and other nonsteroidal anti-inflammatory drugs.
- Most of these individuals are tolerant to weak inhibitors of cyclooxygenase (COX)-1 such as acetaminophen and to preferential and selective inhibitors of COX-2.
- The mechanisms of urticaria and angioedema induced by nonsteroidal anti-inflammatory drugs (NSAIDs) observed in patients with chronic spontaneous urticaria/angioedema involve the inhibition of COX-1.
- Patient management includes avoidance of classic NSAIDs, the use of drugs that do not inhibit COX-1 for symptomatic relief of pain, fever, and inflammation, and the pharmacologic treatment of chronic urticaria.

## INTRODUCTION

Nonsteroidal anti-inflammatory drugs (NSAIDs) are a chemically heterogeneous group of substances that interfere with inflammatory processes by blocking the function of a group of enzymes called cyclooxygenases. Under physiologic conditions, arachidonic acid (AA) derived from cell membrane phospholipids by the action of phospholipases is metabolized to produce potent inflammatory mediators through 2 major pathways. The first of these is the cyclooxygenase (COX) pathway, which participates in the conversion of AA into prostaglandins and thromboxanes. The second is the lipoxygenase pathway.

There are 2 COX isoforms, COX-1 and COX-2. COX-1 is the constitutive isoenzyme, which is present in all cells, and whose actions are inhibited by aspirin

Department of Allergy and Clinical Immunology, Centro Médico-Docente La Trinidad, Carretera La Trinidad-El Hatillo, Caracas, Venezuela
* Correspondence author. Sexta transversal *Urbanización* Altamira, piso 8, consultorio 803, Caracas 1060, Venezuela.
*E-mail address:* sanchezbmario@gmail.com

Immunol Allergy Clin N Am 33 (2013) 251–262
http://dx.doi.org/10.1016/j.iac.2012.10.004
0889-8561/13/$ – see front matter © 2013 Elsevier Inc. All rights reserved.
immunology.theclinics.com

(acetylsalicylic acid or ASA) and all classic NSAIDs. COX-2, the inducible isoform, is present exclusively in inflammatory and immune cells, is upregulated after stimulation by cytokines, growth factors, bacterial lipopolysaccharides, tumor promoters, and other factors, and is inhibited by the classic NSAIDs and also by the new preferential (nimesulide, meloxicam) and selective (coxibs) COX-2 inhibitors. The second metabolic route for AA is the 5-lipoxygenase (5-LO) pathway, which converts AA to cysteinyl leukotrienes (LTC4, LTD4, and LTE4).

Hypersensitivity reactions to NSAIDs are a major cause of morbidity worldwide. Most studies show that reactions to aspirin and NSAIDs are the second leading cause of drug hypersensitivity reactions, after antibiotics (especially β-lactams), for hospitalized as well as ambulatory patients.[1]

Recently the European Network of Drug Allergy (ENDA), the Interest Group on Drug Hypersensitivity of the European Academy of Allergy and Clinical Immunology (EAACI), and the European Network on Hypersensitivity to Aspirin and NSAIDs (HANNA) proposed an updated classification of hypersensitivity reactions to NSAIDs based on timing of initiation, clinical picture, and pharmacologic pattern of the reaction. There were at least 2 previous articles that proposed for the first time a systematic understanding of the various clinical and pharmacologic patterns of reactions induced by NSAIDs.[2,3] In the new classification, reactions to NSAIDs are divided into immediate (occurring after minutes to several hours of drug exposure) and delayed (appearing more than 24 hours after drug intake).[4]

Aspirin-exacerbated cutaneous disease (AECD) is characterized by flares of urticaria and angioedema induced by aspirin and other NSAIDs in patients who suffer chronic spontaneous urticaria. This picture should be distinguished from acute cross-reactive urticaria and angioedema occurring in patients who are otherwise healthy, which is now designated as urticaria and angioedema induced by multiple NSAIDs.[5]

## PHARMACOLOGIC OVERVIEW OF NSAIDS

As previously mentioned, AA is metabolized to produce potent inflammatory mediators by 2 enzymatic pathways: the COX and the 5-LO pathways. NSAIDs are a group of medications that antagonize inflammation by interfering with the function of cyclooxygenases. The inhibition of COX-1 results in a shunting of AA metabolism toward the 5-LO pathway, with enhancement of the production of cysteinyl leukotrienes.

Aspirin and the classic NSAIDs inhibit both COX isoforms, COX-1 and COX-2, whereas the new preferential (nimesulide, meloxicam) and selective (coxibs: rofecoxib, etoricoxib, valdecoxib, parecoxib, lumiracoxib) COX-2 inhibitors do not interfere with (or inhibit weakly) COX-1, and are better tolerated by the gastrointestinal tract because they do not reduce significantly the synthesis of prostaglandin $E_2$ in the stomach.

Recently, new COX isoenzymes that are preferentially inhibited by acetaminophen, pyrazolones, and antipyrine have been described as COX-1 variants and designated COX-2b and COX-3.[6,7] In **Box 1**, a classification of NSAIDs according to their COX inhibitory properties is presented.

## ASPIRIN-EXACERBATED CUTANEOUS DISEASE
### Definition and Prevalence

Urticaria is characterized by the sudden appearance of wheals. Wheals are cutaneous swelling of variable size, almost invariably surrounded by a reflex erythema, with associated itching or, sometimes, a burning sensation of transient nature, with the skin

---

**Box 1**
**Classification of NSAIDs according to their selectivity for COX isoenzymes**

Weak COX inhibitors

Acetaminophen, pyrazolone, salsalate

Inhibitors of COX-1 and COX-2

Piroxicam, indomethacin, sulindac, tolmetin, ibuprofen, naproxen, penoprofen, meclofenamate, mefenamic acid, diflunisal, ketoprofen, diclofenac, ketorolac, etodolac, nabumetone, oxaprozin, flurbiprofen

Preferential COX-2 inhibitors

Nimesulide, meloxicam

Selective COX-2 inhibitors

Celecoxib, rofecoxib, valdecoxib, etoricoxib, parecoxib, lumiracoxib

---

returning to its normal appearance in 1 to 24 hours. Angioedema can be defined as a sudden and pronounced swelling of the deep dermis and subcutaneous tissue or mucous membranes, with a painful rather than an itching sensation, and a slower resolution rate (up to 72 hours).[8,9]

Urticaria and angioedema are classified according to their duration into acute (less than 6 weeks) and chronic (longer than 6 weeks), and are classed as spontaneous and inducible on the basis of the presence or absence of inducing factors.[8]

Two subsets of patients who develop cross-reactive urticaria and/or angioedema during placebo-controlled oral challenges with aspirin or NSAIDs have been described.[10] First, NSAIDs may cause acute episodes of urticaria/angioedema in cross-reactive patients only when exposed to the drug.[11] These patients do not have chronic idiopathic urticaria, belong to the group designated as multiple NSAID-induced urticaria, and are the focus of an article elsewhere in this issue.[4]

On the other hand, aspirin and NSAIDs may also aggravate preexisting chronic spontaneous urticaria/angioedema.[12–16] Analogous to aspirin-exacerbated respiratory disease (AERD), this condition has been designated as aspirin-exacerbated cutaneous disease or AECD, to denote that chronic urticaria evolves independently of the intake of aspirin and NSAIDs, and that those drugs are not the cause but the exacerbating factor for the hives.[5] In fact, from 21% to 30% of patients with chronic spontaneous urticaria (CSU) develop hives after receiving NSAIDs,[17] with active CSU increasing the risk of reacting to NSAIDs.[18] Furthermore, Asero[15] observed that the reaction to aspirin/NSAIDs may precede the onset of episodes of chronic urticaria. This observation means that some patients classified as being normal actually have latent chronic idiopathic urticaria, which is temporarily exacerbated by NSAIDs, long before the disease declares itself.

Patients with AECD react to drugs that exert an inhibitory effect on COX-1 and generally are tolerant to selective COX-2 inhibitors.[19,20] A genetic predisposition for cutaneous NSAID hypersensitivity may play a role in AECD, because various investigators have observed the association between various genetic polymorphisms and this disease.[21,22]

## Pathogenesis

CSU and angioedema, previously known as chronic idiopathic urticaria, are characterized by the recurrent appearance of wheals or subcutaneous tissue edema lasting longer than 6 weeks. Other forms of chronic urticaria that should be distinguished from CSU are the inducible urticarias such as those induced by physical agents (cold, pressure, heat, sunlight, vibration, aquagenic) and other inducible urticarias such as cholinergic, contact, and exercise-induced urticaria.[8]

Although the mechanisms of CSU are not completely understood, chronic inflammation of the skin and deep dermis with the release of several inflammatory mediators is responsible for the cutaneous swelling, generally surrounded by erythema, and the itching/burning sensation characteristic of the wheals. In most patients there is no identifiable exogenous stimulus leading to the production of hives, although in some patients nonspecific environmental triggers such as exercise, climatic changes, and emotional stress are present.

Different hypotheses have been postulated to explain the mechanisms involved in CSU, including psychosomatic factors, food and additive intolerance or allergy, autoreactivity or autoimmunity, and poorly understood disturbances of basophils and immunoglobulin E (IgE).

Patients with chronic urticaria associated with aspirin-induced urticaria/angioedema react to various NSAIDs that have a different chemical composition but share the ability to inhibit COX-1. Usually they are tolerant to COX-2 inhibitors.[20,23]

The mechanisms responsible for the production of aspirin/NSAID-induced exacerbations of chronic urticaria and angioedema involve the inhibition of COX-1, as demonstrated by Mastalerz and colleagues.[24] These investigators observed that patients with CSU who experience disease exacerbations when exposed to aspirin have increased basal levels of urinary LTE4 (uLTE4) when compared with aspirintolerant CSU patients. Further increases of uLTE4 occur in the group of aspirinsensitive patients after oral aspirin challenge. It is postulated that the inhibition of COX-1 by NSAIDs results in a decreased prostaglandin production, enhanced inflammatory mediator release in the skin, and symptoms.[25] Because leukotriene receptor antagonists are able to inhibit these reactions, it is likely that the increased cysteinyl leukotriene production contributes to the inflammatory process.[26,27]

It is presently accepted that chronic urticaria is associated with autoimmune diseases, especially chronic autoimmune thyroiditis.[28] Furthermore, 5% to 10% of patients with CSU have circulating immunoglobulin G (IgG) anti-IgE, which is functional and induces mediator release from mast cells and basophils on cross-linking of receptor-bound IgE,[29] and 30% to 40% of patients have IgG antibody to the $\alpha$ subunit of the high-affinity IgE receptor itself.[30] The presence of these circulating autoantibodies is usually demonstrated by means of an autologous intradermal skin test with the patient's serum or plasma.

The presence of positive autologous serum and plasma skin tests suggests an association between CSU, autoimmunity, and aspirin hypersensitivity.[16,31] Another interesting observation has been recently reported by Ye and colleagues,[32] who observed an association between IgE immune response to toxic shock syndrome toxin (TSST)-1 and aspirin sensitivity in patients with chronic urticaria.

A genetic predisposition for NSAID cutaneous hypersensitivity has been observed in various populations, and polymorphisms of HLA antigens (HLA-DRB1*1302 and HLA-DB1*069), neutrophil-related genes, LTC4 synthase, 5-LO, FcεRI, and histamine N-methyltransferase have been suggested as genetic markers for NSAID-induced urticaria/angioedema.[21,22,33–35]

## Clinical Picture

In AECD wheals and/or angioedema usually appear after 1 to 4 hours of drug administration, but in case an injectable form of the drug (eg, ketoprofen or dipyrone) is administered by the parenteral route the clinical picture may begin earlier and be more severe. Rarely late reactions can occur. Individual hives tend to disappear within a few hours but may persist for several days.

Prognostic factors for longer duration and increased severity of CSU are the presence of concomitant angioedema, positivity of autologous serum skin test, and comorbidity with physical urticaria.

Quiralte and colleagues[11] reported that the most common clinical presentation of cutaneous NSAID hypersensitivity is eyelid (periorbital) angioedema. To illustrate the clinical presentation of patients with AECD, 2 cases are described in **Boxes 2** and **3**.

It is unusual that AERD and AECD coexist in the same patient, and these 2 phenotypes are generally regarded as different clinical entities. However, Isik and colleagues[36] observed that in some patients asthma and nasal polyposis may co-occur in patients with CSU and NSAID hypersensitivity, although it should be emphasized that this association is rarely present.

## Diagnosis

A medical history and physical examination are helpful to establish the diagnosis of chronic urticaria. Recurrent wheals with or without angioedema lasting for more than 6 weeks, usually in the absence of precipitating factors, are typically associated with CSU, and initial complementary studies are oriented to rule out concomitant systemic diseases and the presence of triggering or exacerbating factors. Present guidelines suggest performing a set of screening tests that includes a differential blood count, liver function tests, erythrocyte sedimentation rate, and C-reactive protein. An explicit recommendation in the guidelines is to inquire early specifically about drug intake temporarily associated with cutaneous symptoms, and more especially about NSAIDs.[8]

---

**Box 2**
**Case report**

A 42-year-old male patient was referred to the Allergology clinics in January 2011 after complaining of eyelid and lip edema appearing 2 hours after the ingestion of ibuprofen, 400 mg, which was taken for toothache. During the medical interrogation the patient reported having recurrent tongue and facial edema for the last 4 years without any identifiable triggering agent, and palpebral angioedema induced by sodium diclofenac. Prednisone, 50 mg every day for 5 days and fexofenadine, 180 mg for 1 month were indicated.

Two months later the patient returned to the emergency room because of eyelid edema and cough (**Fig. 1**). Treatment with intravenous hydrocortisone, 100 mg and chlorpheniramine, 10 mg were given, and at the time of discharge prednisone, 50 mg for 5 days and cetirizine, 10 mg for 1 month were prescribed.

*Laboratory investigations* done on March 3, 2011: Complement: $CH_{50}$ 113.5 units/mL. C3 133 mg/dL. C4 38.3 mg/dL. Hematologic values and blood chemistry: within normal limits. Stools: cysts of *Giardia lamblia*.

*Treatment:* (1) Cetirizine 10 mg every day for 3 months. (2) Nitazoxanide 500 mg twice a day for 3 days. (3) Avoidance of NSAIDs that inhibit COX-1. (4) Acetaminophen for mild pain or fever. Celecoxib for inflammation or moderate to severe pain.

*Diagnosis:* (1) Chronic angioedema. (2) AECD. (3) Giardiasis.

*Comments:* No confirmatory provocation tests were considered pertinent for this patient because the history was clearly indicative of chronic spontaneous angioedema aggravated by 2 cross-reacting NSAIDs. Oral challenges with acetaminophen and celecoxib were tolerated.

> **Box 3**
> **Case report**
>
> A 28-year-old male patient consulted because he had recurrent itchy wheals predominantly on the lower limbs for 8 years, with increased frequency and severity for the last 6 weeks (**Fig. 2**). The skin lesions were occasionally accompanied by lip edema.
>
> The patient referred that the wheals increased after taking analgesics, including aspirin and dipyrone. There were no other previous or current significant medical problems.
>
> Routine *laboratory* investigations included hematological tests, erythrosedimentation rate, blood chemistry, urinalysis, and coprologic evaluation. All resulted negative or within normal ranges.
>
> *Management:* (1) Levocetirizine 5 mg every day. (2) Prednisone 50 mg every day for 6 days. (3) Avoidance of classic NSAIDs. (4) Alternative drugs for pain, fever, and inflammation: acetaminophen or meloxicam.
>
> *Diagnosis:* CSU/angioedema exacerbated by NSAIDs (AECD).
>
> *Comments:* A test for tolerance is recommended to make sure that alternative NSAIDs can be used with safety in these patients. It has been observed that if doses of alternative NSAIDs are increased (eg, >1000 mg of acetaminophen), cutaneous reactions may occur.

Patient questioning and examination may provide information for further testing to investigate infectious diseases (for example, *Helicobacter pylori*, parasites), in vivo or in vitro tests for IgE-mediated allergy to environmental or food allergens, autoantibodies (including thyroid antibodies), tests for thyroid function, and specific tests for physical urticarias. Intradermal tests with autologous serum or plasma allow the confirmation of mast cell–activating autoantibodies (anti-FcRεl or anti-IgE) or other serum factors able to induce mediator release in the skin, and to confirm CSU-associated autoimmunity or autoreactivity. Skin biopsy is generally indicated only for differential diagnosis from other skin diseases, and especially from urticarial vasculitis.

AECD can be suspected from questioning the patient, because frequently the patient will refer a history of chronic spontaneous hives or angioedema accompanied

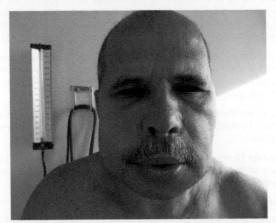

**Fig. 1.** A 42-year-old male patient with chronic angioedema and aspirin-exacerbated cutaneous disease (AECD). Observe the diffuse angioedema of the face, bilateral eyelid, and upper and lower lip.

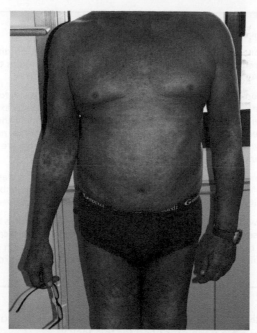

**Fig. 2.** A 28-year-old male patient with chronic spontaneous urticaria and angioedema, and NSAID hypersensitivity (AECD) is shown. Observe the presence of generalized urticaria, which involves upper and lower limbs and the trunk.

by repeated exacerbations of urticaria/angioedema after taking different COX-1 inhibitors. When the relation between skin symptoms and NSAID administration is unclear, oral provocation tests with aspirin using standard protocols are useful to confirm AECD (**Table 1**).[5] These challenges should not be performed during urticarial exacerbations, and are better done after at least 1 to 2 weeks during which the patient does not show any skin eruption.[37] The provocation test should be performed without interrupting the current treatment of chronic urticaria to avoid false-positive results due to reactivation of the underlying disease when therapy is discontinued (**Box 4**).

Other NSAIDs can be tested in a similar form, using protocols available in the literature.[38] There is no in vitro test presently validated for routine diagnosis of cutaneous

| Table 1 | | | |
| --- | --- | --- | --- |
| Single-blind oral provocation test with acetylsalicylic acid (aspirin; ASA) for patients with urticaria and angioedema | | | |
| **Day 1** | **Day 2** | **Day 3** | **Day 4** |
| Placebo | ASA 100 mg | ASA 325 mg | ASA 650 mg |
| Placebo | ASA 200 mg | | |

On days 1 and 2, doses are administered every 2 hours.
 Skin scores are recorded every 2 hours.
 Treatment of chronic urticaria is continued during the provocation test (for explanation see the section Diagnosis).
 In Europe, the recommended ASA doses for testing are 71 mg, 117 mg, 312 mg, and 500 mg.[37]

---

**Box 4**
**Protocol for oral provocation test with NSAIDs (single- or double-blind)**

Drugs or placebo concealed in identical opaque capsules are given on different days. Drug doses are administered 1 hour apart with a 3-hour observation period in the hospital. Doses for the different NSAIDs are shown in **Table 2**.

Vital signs and pulmonary function (forced expiratory volume in 1 second, forced vital capacity, midexpiratory phase [25%–75%] of forced expiratory flow, and peak expiratory flow) are monitored at baseline and hourly for 3 hours. The skin, nose, eyes, and thorax are examined hourly and the presence of breathlessness, cough, wheezing, dysphonia, nasal or ocular itching, sneezing, rhinorrhea, nasal obstruction, and conjunctival erythema are investigated every hour by physical examination.

For urticaria and angioedema the percentage of skin involved is calculated as follows: head and neck 30%, chest 20%, abdomen 20%, upper limbs 15%, and lower limbs 15%. The test is considered positive if an increase of 20% or more from baseline is observed.

Previous treatment with antihistamines and/or anti-inflammatory drugs is maintained during the test to avoid false positives due to spontaneous exacerbations of urticaria and/or angioedema. The tests are done on an outpatient basis in a medical center with easy availability of medications and equipment required for the treatment of reactions that occur during the challenge.

---

NSAID hypersensitivity, although the basophil activation test and the sulfidoleukotriene release assay have been proposed for this task.[39]

### Management

The treatment of CSU and angioedema is based on preventive measures designed to reduce the effects of provoking and exacerbating factors, and on pharmacologic therapies. These treatments follow the guidelines proposed by international organizations and experts in the area.[40] The first choice is to use second-generation antihistamines in the usually recommended doses. If there is not a satisfactory response, the doses can be increased progressively every 2 weeks up to 4 times the regular dose. Add-on therapy with leukotriene receptor antagonists is the next step if there is no symptom improvement. In patients who do not respond, additional medications include anti-inflammatory, immunosuppressive, and biologic therapies. A new Position Paper on

**Table 2**
**Doses of NSAIDs used for oral provocation tests**

| Drug | Doses (mg) |
| --- | --- |
| Dipyrone | 250, 500 |
| Acetaminophen | 250, 500, 1000 |
| Ibuprofen | 50, 100, 200 |
| Diclofenac | 25, 50 |
| Ketoprofen | 25, 50 |
| Naproxen | 125, 250 |
| Nimesulide | 50, 100 |
| Meloxicam | 7.5, 15 |
| Celecoxib | 100, 200 |
| Rofecoxib | 25, 50 |
| Etoricoxib | 60, 120 |

**Table 3**
**Pharmacologic treatment of chronic urticaria and angioedema based on the quality of scientific evidence**

| Drug | Quality of Evidence | Strength of Recommendation |
|---|---|---|
| Nonsedating antihistamines | High | Strong (f) |
| Sedating antihistamines | High | Strong (a) |
| Increased doses of nonsedating antihistamines | Moderate | Weak (f) |
| Anti-H2 antihistamines | Moderate | Weak (f) |
| Oral corticosteroids (short courses) | Low | Weak (f) |
| Oral corticosteroids | Very low | Strong (a) |
| Leukotriene receptor antagonists (add on) | Low | Weak (f) |
| Anti-inflammatory agents: Dapsone Sulfasalazine Hydroxychloroquine Colchicine Mycophenolate mofetil | Low to very low | Weak (f) |
| Immunosuppressive agents: | | |
| Cyclosporin A | Moderate | Weak (f) |
| Methotrexate | Very low | Weak (f) |
| Cyclophosphamide | Very low | Weak (f) |
| Biologic agents: | | |
| Omalizumab | Moderate | Weak (f) |
| Intravenous immunoglobulin | Low | Weak (f) |

For cyclosporin A and omalizumab, the recommendation is stronger than for other immunosuppressive, anti-inflammatory or biologic therapies.

(f): recommendation for. (a): recommendation against.

*Data from* Sánchez-Borges M, Asero R, Ansotegui IJ, et al. World Allergy Organization position paper. Diagnosis and treatment of urticaria and angioedema—a worldwide perspective. World Allergy Organ J 2012;5:125–47.

the diagnosis and treatment of urticaria and angioedema of the World Allergy Organization presents therapeutic recommendations for urticaria and angioedema based on the grading of efficacy according to evidence-based medicine (**Table 3**).[41] Out of presently available therapies for recalcitrant patients with CSU, cyclosporine A and omalizumab appear to deliver the best results when compared with the other drugs (**Box 5**).[42,43]

---

**Box 5**
**Management of aspirin-exacerbated cutaneous disease**

- Avoidance of COX-1 inhibitors
- Weak COX-1 inhibitors (acetaminophen) for fever or mild pain
- Preferential COX-2 inhibitors (nimesulide, meloxicam) for pain and inflammation
- Selective COX-2 inhibitors (coxibs: rofecoxib, etoricob, celecoxib) for pain and inflammation
- Desensitization not usually recommended
- Management of CSU and angioedema as per guidelines[40]

Avoidance of aspirin and classic NSAIDs is indicated for patients with AECD, but analogous to AERD the underlying chronic urticaria is not affected by drug elimination. All COX-1 inhibitors should not be prescribed, and alternative weak COX-1 inhibitors (acetaminophen) or preferential and selective inhibitors of COX-2 (nimesulide, meloxicam, coxibs), which are tolerated by most AECD patients, can be used for relief of pain, fever, and inflammation. Provocation tests are performed to confirm tolerance to these alternative anti-inflammatory drugs.[19,23,44,45]

Aspirin desensitization, as used in patients with AERD, is not generally indicated for patients with cross-reactive aspirin-induced urticaria and angioedema, because persistent aspirin-induced hives are routine and desensitization almost never occurs (Table 3).[46]

## SUMMARY

About one-third of patients with CSU and angioedema who receive aspirin or the classic NSAIDs show exacerbation of their cutaneous disease. Most of these subjects can tolerate weak COX-1 inhibitors such as acetaminophen and inhibitors of COX-2.

The mechanisms of aspirin/NSAID-induced urticaria and angioedema observed in patients with chronic urticaria involve the inhibition of COX-1. Patient management includes avoidance of classic NSAIDs, use of non–COX-1 inhibitor NSAIDs for symptomatic relief of pain, fever, and inflammation, and pharmacologic treatment of chronic urticaria according to presently available guidelines.

## REFERENCES

1. Gomes CR, Demoly P. Epidemiology of hypersensitivity drug reactions. Curr Opin Allergy Clin Immunol 2005;5:309–16.
2. Stevenson D. Challenge procedures in detection of reactions to aspirin and nonsteroidal anti-inflammatory drugs. Ann Allergy 1993;71:117–8.
3. Stevenson DD, Sánchez-Borges M, Szczeklik A. Classification of allergic and pseudoallergic reactions to drugs that inhibit cyclo-oxygenase enzymes. Ann Allergy Asthma Immunol 2001;87:1–4.
4. Kowalski ML, Makowska JS, Blanca M, et al. Hypersensitivity to nonsteroidal anti-inflammatory drugs (NSAIDs)—classification, diagnosis and management: review of the EAACI/ENDA and GA2LEN/HANNA. Allergy 2011;66:818–29.
5. Sánchez-Borges M. NSAID hypersensitivity (respiratory, cutaneous, and generalized anaphylactic symptoms). Med Clin North Am 2010;94:853–64.
6. Chandrasekharan NV, Dai H, Roos KL, et al. COX-3 a cyclooxygenase-1 variant inhibited by acetaminophen and other analgesic/antipyretic drugs: cloning, structure and expression. Proc Natl Acad Sci U S A 2002;99:13926–31.
7. Simmons DL, Botting RM, Robertson PM, et al. Induction of an acetaminophen-sensitive cyclooxygenase with reduced sensitivity to nonsteroidal anti-inflammatory drugs. Proc Natl Acad Sci U S A 1999;96:3275–80.
8. Zuberbier T, Asero R, Bindslev-Jensen C, et al. EAACI/GA2LEN/EDF/WAO guideline: definition, classification and diagnosis of urticaria. Allergy 2009;64:1417–26.
9. Kaplan A. Clinical practice. Chronic urticaria and angioedema. N Engl J Med 2002;346:175–9.
10. Quiralte J, Blanco C, Delgado J, et al. Challenge-based clinical patterns of 223 Spanish patients with nonsteroidal anti-inflammatory-drug-induced reactions. J Investig Allergol Clin Immunol 2007;17:182–8.

11. Quiralte J, Blanco C, Castillo R, et al. Intolerance to non-steroidal anti-inflammatory drugs: results of controlled drug challenges in 98 patients. J Allergy Clin Immunol 1996;98:678–85.
12. Moore-Robinson M, Warin RP. Effect of salicylates in urticaria. Br Med J 1967;4: 262–4.
13. Settipane RA, Constantine HP, Settipane GA. Aspirin intolerance and recurrent urticaria in normal adults and children. Allergy 1980;35:149–54.
14. Grattan CE. Aspirin sensitivity and urticaria. Clin Exp Dermatol 2003;28:123–7.
15. Asero R. Intolerance to nonsteroidal anti-inflammatory drugs might precede by years the onset of chronic urticaria. J Allergy Clin Immunol 2003;111:1095–8.
16. Erbagci Z. Multiple NSAID intolerance in chronic idiopathic urticaria is correlated with delayed, pronounced and prolonged autoreactivity. J Dermatol 2004;31: 376–82.
17. Doeglas HM. Reactions to aspirin and food additives in patients with chronic urticaria, including the physical urticarias. Br J Dermatol 1975;93:135–44.
18. Mastalerz L, Setkowicz M, Szczeklik A. A mechanism of chronic urticaria exacerbation by aspirin. Curr Allergy Asthma Rep 2005;5:277–83.
19. Zembowicz A, Mastalerz L, Setkowicz M, et al. Safety of cyclooxygenase 2 inhibitors and increased leukotriene synthesis in chronic urticaria with sensitivity to nonsteroidal anti-inflammatory drugs. Arch Dermatol 2003;139:1577–82.
20. Asero R. Etoricoxib challenge in patients with chronic urticaria with NSAID intolerance. Clin Exp Dermatol 2007;32:661–3.
21. Bae JS, Kim SH, Ye YM, et al. Significant association of FcεRIα promoter polymorphisms with aspirin-intolerant chronic urticaria. J Allergy Clin Immunol 2007;119: 449–56.
22. Kim SH, Ye YM, Palikhe NS, et al. Genetic and ethnic risk factors associated with drug hypersensitivity. Curr Opin Allergy Clin Immunol 2010;10:280–90.
23. Sánchez-Borges M, Capriles-Hulett A, Caballero-Fonseca F, et al. Tolerability to new COX-2 inhibitors in NSAID-sensitive patients with cutaneous reactions. Ann Allergy Asthma Immunol 2001;87:201–4.
24. Mastalerz L, Setkowicz M, Sanak M, et al. Hypersensitivity to aspirin: common eicosanoid alterations in urticaria and asthma. J Allergy Clin Immunol 2004; 113:771–5.
25. Setkowicz M, Mastalerz L, Podolec-Rubis M, et al. Clinical course and urinary eicosanoids in patients with aspirin-induced urticaria followed up for 4 years. J Allergy Clin Immunol 2009;123:174–8.
26. Perez C, Sánchez-Borges M, Suárez-Chacón R. Pretreatment with montelukast blocks NSAID-induced urticaria and angioedema. J Allergy Clin Immunol 2001; 108:1060–1.
27. Asero R. Leukotriene receptor antagonists may prevent NSAID-induced exacerbations in patients with chronic urticaria. Ann Allergy Asthma Immunol 2000;85: 156–7.
28. Leznoff A, Josse RG, Denburg J, et al. Association of chronic urticaria and angioedema with thyroid autoimmunity. Arch Dermatol 1983;119(8):636–40.
29. Gruber B, Baeza M, Marchese M, et al. Prevalence and functional role of anti-IgE autoantibodies in urticarial syndromes. J Invest Dermatol 1988;90:213–7.
30. Hide M, Francis D, Grattan C, et al. Autoantibodies against the high-affinity IgE receptor as a cause of histamine release in chronic urticaria. N Engl J Med 1993;328:1599–604.
31. Asero R. Predictive value of autologous plasma skin test for multiple nonsteroidal anti-inflammatory drug intolerance. Int Arch Allergy Immunol 2007;144:226–30.

32. Ye YM, Hur GY, Park HJ, et al. Association of specific IgE to staphylococcal superantigens with the phenotype of chronic urticaria. J Korean Med Sci 2008; 23:845–51.

33. Pacor ML, Di Lorenzo G, Mansueto P, et al. Relationship between human leukocyte antigen class I and class II and chronic idiopathic urticaria associated with aspirin and/or NSAID hypersensitivity. Mediat Inflamm 2006;1–5 article ID 62489.

34. Kim SY, Park HS. Genetic markers for differentiating aspirin hypersensitivity. Yonsei Med J 2006;47:15–21.

35. Sánchez-Borges M, Acevedo N, Vergara C, et al. The A-444C polymorphism in the leukotriene C4 synthase gene is associated with aspirin-induced urticaria. J Investig Allergol Clin Immunol 2009;19:375–82.

36. Isik SR, Karakaya G, Celikel S, et al. Association between asthma, rhinitis and NSAID hypersensitivity in chronic urticaria patients and prevalence rates. Int Arch Allergy Immunol 2009;150:299–306.

37. Nizankowska-Mogilnicka E, Bochenek G, Mastalerz L, et al. EAACI/GA2LEN guideline: aspirin provocation tests for diagnosis of aspirin hypersensitivity. Allergy 2007;62:1111–8.

38. Messaad D, Sahla H, Benahmed S, et al. Drug provocation tests in patients with a history suggesting an immediate drug hypersensitivity reaction. Ann Intern Med 2004;140:1001–6.

39. Sanz ML, Gamboa P, De Weck AL. A new combined test with flow cytometric basophil activation and determination of sulfidoleukotrienes is useful for in vitro diagnosis of hypersensitivity to aspirin and other nonsteroidal anti-inflammatory drugs. Int Arch Allergy Immunol 2005;136:58–72.

40. Zuberbier T, Asero R, Bindslev-Jensen C, et al. EAACI/GA2LEN/EDF/WAO guideline: management of urticaria. Allergy 2009;64:1427–43.

41. Sánchez-Borges M, Asero R, Ansotegui IJ, et al. World Allergy Organization position paper. Diagnosis and treatment of urticaria and angioedema—a worldwide perspective. World Allergy Organ J 2012; in press.

42. Saini S, Rosen KE, Hsieh HJ, et al. A randomized, placebo-controlled, dose-ranging study of single-dose omalizumab in patients with H(1)-antihistamine-refractory chronic idiopathic urticaria. J Allergy Clin Immunol 2011;128:567–73.

43. Kessel A, Toubi E. Cyclosporine-a in severe chronic urticaria: the option for long-term therapy. Allergy 2010;65:1478–82.

44. Sánchez-Borges M, Caballero-Fonseca F, Capriles-Hulett A. Tolerance of nonsteroidal anti-inflammatory drug-sensitive patients to the highly specific cyclooxygenase 2 inhibitors rofecoxib and valdecoxib. Ann Allergy Asthma Immunol 2005; 94:34–8.

45. Sánchez-Borges M, Caballero-Fonseca F, Capriles-Hulett A. Safety of etoricoxib, a new cyclooxygenase 2 inhibitor, in patients with nonsteroidal anti-inflammatory drug-induced urticaria and angioedema. Ann Allergy Asthma Immunol 2005;95: 154–8.

46. Simon RA. Prevention and treatment of reactions to NSAIDs. Clin Rev Allergy Immunol 2003;24:189–98.

# Cardiovascular Prophylaxis and Aspirin "Allergy"

Katharine M. Woessner, MD*, Ronald A. Simon, MD

## KEYWORDS

- Coronary artery disease • Aspirin-exacerbated respiratory disease
- Cyclooxygenase • Acetylsalicylic acid • Nonsteroidal anti-inflammatory drug

## KEY POINTS

- With rare exceptions, patients with a history of "aspirin/nonsteroidal anti-inflammatory allergy" will be able to safely take aspirin after either graded dose challenge or desensitization.
- Aspirin therapy should not be routinely denied to patients with history of aspirin sensitivity.
- Allergists should be proactive and consistent in their message that aspirin challenge/desensitization can be performed in the acute setting when clinically essential.

Aspirin (acetylsalicylic acid) is a potent antiplatelet therapy and is a cornerstone in the management of coronary artery disease (CAD) and other thrombotic diseases. Aspirin is an inhibitor of cyclooxygenase (COX). In the platelet, irreversible inhibition of COX leads to inhibition of thromboxane-mediated platelet aggregation (**Fig. 1**). A meta-analysis of multiple trials looking at patients at high risk for thrombotic events showed that aspirin is protective in most types of patients at increased risk of occlusive vascular events, including those with an acute myocardial infarction or ischemic stroke, unstable or stable angina, previous myocardial infarction, stroke or cerebral ischemia, peripheral arterial disease, or atrial fibrillation.[1] Despite extensive data supporting the role of aspirin in vascular disease, several at risk patients often fail to receive adequate antiplatelet therapy due to possible allergy to aspirin.

Aspirin therapy can result in a 33% event-reduction rate and is recommended for both primary prevention for at-risk patients and secondary prevention for those who already have cardiovascular disease.[1] Guidelines from the American College of Cardiology (ACC) and the American Heart Association (AHA) cite a class I indication for aspirin therapy unless a true sensitivity to aspirin or nonsteroidal anti-inflammatory drugs (NSAIDs) exists, in which case thienopyridines (clopidogrel, ticagrelor, and

Disclosures: None.
Division of Allergy, Asthma and Immunology, Scripps Clinic, 3811 Valley Centre Drive, San Diego, CA 92130, USA
* Corresponding author.
E-mail address: Woessner.katharine@scrippshealth.org

Immunol Allergy Clin N Am 33 (2013) 263–274
http://dx.doi.org/10.1016/j.iac.2012.11.004
0889-8561/13/$ – see front matter © 2013 Elsevier Inc. All rights reserved.

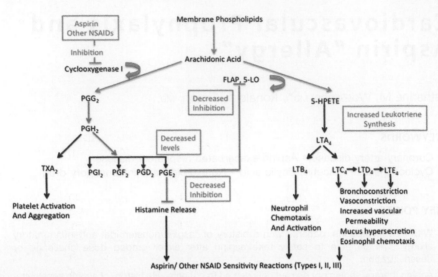

**Fig. 1.** Arachidonic acid is the substrate used to generate prostanoids and leukotrienes (LT). The cyclooxygenase-1 (COX-1) enzyme is the site of inhibition by aspirin and NSAIDs. Activation of COX-1 leads to synthesis of thromboxanes (TXA), a potent activation of platelets, and platelet aggregation, as well as the prostaglandins ($PGI_2$, $PGF_2$, $PGD_2$, and $PGE_2$). Inhibition of COX-1 leads to a rapid depletion of $PGE_2$. In the absence of the braking effect of $PGE_2$ on 5-lipooxygenase (5-LO) and 5-lipoxygenase–activating protein (FLAP), there is a dramatic increase in the synthesis of the cysteinyl leukotrienes. These arachidonic acid metabolites lead to the clinical manifestations of aspirin sensitivity including AERD, urticaria, and angioedema. 5-HPETE, 5-hydroxyperoxyeicosatetraenoic acid.

prasugrel) are alternative antiplatelet agents that can be used.[2,3] Combination therapy for aspirin with clopidogrel reduces adverse cardiovascular events in unstable angina, non–ST-segment elevation myocardial infarction, and ST-segment elevation myocardial infarction.[4,5] It also improves survival and reduces adverse cardiac events in patients with acute coronary syndrome treated with either bare-metal stents (BMS) or drug-eluting stents (DES).[3,5–7] The ACC, AHA, and the Society for Cardiovascular Angiography and Intervention (SCAI) recommend combination therapy for patients with acute coronary syndrome undergoing percutaneous intervention.[3,8] According to the guidelines, therapy with aspirin should be life-long in these patients with CAD.

In the case of aspirin or NSAID hypersensitivity, monotherapy with a thienopyridine may be used as an alternative. However, this is not as cost-effective and carries a risk of hematologic complications including thrombotic thrombocytopenic purpura and neutropenia.[9] An additional concern is the patient who needs to undergo coronary artery bypass grafting (CABG) surgery. Aspirin therapy can be continued through to surgery, whereas other antiplatelet therapies need to be stopped 5 to 7 days before CABG because their continued use is associated with increased CABG-related bleeding. Thus, patients relying on these alternative antiplatelet therapies are at risk of major cardiac events in the 5 to 7 days before surgery, owing to the lack of antiplatelet therapy.

For the physician, facing therapeutic decisions in a patient with cardiovascular disease and aspirin hypersensitivity is complicated, as aspirin/NSAID hypersensitivity can affect up to 0.5% to 1.9% of the general population and can be manifested by aspirin-exacerbated respiratory disease (AERD), urticaria/angioedema, or anaphylaxis.[10–12] The prevalence of AERD is estimated to be 4.3 % to 11% of asthmatics by history or review of medical records, and may be as high as 21% when aspirin challenges are used for diagnosis.[13,14] For aspirin-induced urticarial/angioedema the prevalence upward of 0.3% in the general population.[10] In patients with chronic urticaria, approximately one-third will experience an exacerbation with the use of COX-1–inhibiting NSAIDs and aspirin.[15] Alternatively, the listed aspirin allergy on the medical record may be aspirin-induced gastritis, tinnitus, or misdiagnosis with aspirin as an innocent bystander.

Given the demonstrated efficacy of aspirin in cardiovascular disease, what should one do when faced with a patient who has an allergy to aspirin? Many patients erroneously believe they are allergic to aspirin and can be identified by taking a careful history to determine that their "allergy" was either a side effect or other misattribution to aspirin. Other patients who are allergic to a single NSAID have erroneously been counseled to avoid all NSAIDs including aspirin, whereas others are at risk of urticaria and/or angioedema with all COX-1–inhibiting NSAIDs including aspirin may not be aware of cross-sensitization. These clinical decisions are difficult for allergy specialists, and frequently even more daunting for practicing cardiology and neurology specialists. For those who report a prior reaction to aspirin, options such as aspirin challenge and desensitization are available and are recommended in the various cardiology guidelines.[16] The focus of this article on providing a practical approach to the patient with a history of aspirin hypersensitivity who needs aspirin therapy.

The first issue to be addressed is identifying the type of reaction to aspirin the patient has previously experienced. This process is critical, as it will dictate subsequent intervention. The various types of reactions are listed here.

Type I: Aspirin-exacerbated respiratory disease. AERD is a unique disease whereby reactions to NSAIDs or aspirin occur in conjunction with sinus disease, nasal polyps, and asthma. Although asthma is not always present, nasal polyps and sinus disease exist in nearly all patients. These patients will typically experience worsening nasal and ocular symptoms as well as asthma symptoms within 1 to 2 hours of ingestion of any medication that blocks the COX-1 enzyme. Important historical clues in identifying these patients are the existence of sinus disease, loss of smell, the presence of reactions to more than one COX-1 inhibitor, and a typical reaction involving the airway.[17] During NSAID-induced respiratory reactions, levels of prostaglandin $E_2$ are rapidly depleted. In the absence of the braking effect of prostaglandin $E_2$ on 5-lipoxygenase–activating protein and 5-lipoxygenase, there is a marked increase in cysteinyl leukotriene synthesis and release, along with release of histamine from mast cells (see **Fig. 1**). With few exceptions, all patients with AERD can undergo successful aspirin desensitization.

Type II: Urticaria/angioedema in the setting of chronic urticaria (CIU). NSAIDs can cause worsening urticaria and angioedema in patients who have active CIU. These patients likely have a history of tolerating NSAIDs or aspirin, but in the midst of their chronic urticaria have worsening of urticaria from the mast cell–destabilizing properties of NSAIDs. These patients will have a history of persistent urticaria made worse by NSAIDs and likely have a history of tolerance of NSAIDs during remission of their underlying urticaria. The proposed pathophysiology, similar to that of AERD, is related to COX-1 inhibition leading to excessive leukotriene production by 5-lipoxygenase activity, and thus to increased vascular permeability and subsequent urticaria.[18] The Scripps experience has been that these patients cannot be desensitized to aspirin during the active phase of their chronic urticaria. This COX-1–mediated effect will occur with any NSAID or aspirin. The prevalence of NSAID-induced urticarial in patients with chronic urticaria is between 20% and 30%.[19,20] Therefore, it is worth challenging a patient with chronic urticaria because up to two-thirds will tolerate aspirin.

*Type III: Urticaria and angioedema induced by multiple NSAIDs mediated through COX-1 inhibition.* These patients do not have preexisting urticaria and also have no evidence of nasal polyps or asthma. As expected by the mechanism, they may have experienced urticaria or angioedema from several members of the NSAID family. Unlike the patient with underlying chronic urticaria, these patients generally can undergo successful aspirin desensitization.

*Type IV: Single NSAID-induced reactions.* NSAIDs can cause isolated, immunologically mediated urticaria and angioedema and/or anaphylaxis. The presumed mechanism is formation of immunoglobulin E (IgE) antibodies against specific epitopes in specific NSAIDs. These patients will have reactions related to one specific NSAID. These reactions are poorly understood, but the specificity of the reaction to one NSAID suggests that a specific IgE mechanism is involved, possibly attributable to drug haptenization. A history of tolerance of other NSAIDs should highlight this type of reaction as most likely. These reactions are limited to a specific NSAID but, because of structural similarity among a family of NSAIDs, cross-reactions may exist (see the article by Woessner and colleagues elsewhere in this issue on classification of NSAID reactions). Patients with an IgE-mediated reaction to any other NSAID should not have difficulty taking aspirin, whose chemical structure eliminates cross-recognition by specific IgE antibodies.

Aspirin has been reported in the literature as a historical cause of anaphylaxis by patients seen in emergency rooms.[21] There is one report of positive skin tests to lysyl aspirin in patients with aspirin-induced urticaria.[22,23] These observations suggest that aspirin-induced anaphylaxis is a possibility. Nevertheless, despite an extensive literature search and careful review, peer consultation throughout multiple medical systems, and an exhaustive review of the cases of aspirin reactions in the Scripps Medical System, the authors are unable to find even one convincing case of an anaphylactic reaction to aspirin.

## DIAGNOSIS OF ASPIRIN/NSAID HYPERSENSITIVITY

There are no established tests on skin or blood that can reliably diagnose hypersensitivity to aspirin/NSAIDs. As such, provocative challenge tests are the only available modalities in the United States.

## REVIEW OF THE LITERATURE

Because of the often emergent need of aspirin for cardiovascular disease, there is a paucity of literature on well-controlled aspirin challenges/desensitizations in this patient population. Thus, before performing desensitization it is almost always unknown whether the patient even has hypersensitivity to aspirin. The latest study by De Luca and colleagues[24] involved 43 patients with a history suggesting aspirin hypersensitivity who needed cardiac stenting, more than 50% of whom had acute coronary syndrome. The patients underwent a rapid intravenous aspirin challenge/desensitization protocol either before the catheterization, in the catheterization laboratory, or following the procedure. A success rate of 97.6% was reported. One patient with chronic urticaria did not tolerate aspirin therapy. McMullan and Wedner[25] have recently published a retrospective study looking at 81 patients with reported aspirin allergy and cardiovascular disease who underwent aspirin desensitization, including 22 treated as outpatients. The investigators noted that 19.7% of the desensitizations were associated with reactions, with 5 patients unable to complete the aspirin desensitization. Risk factors for reactions during desensitization included history of aspirin-induced angioedema and historical reaction to aspirin within the previous year.

A variety of other experiences with desensitization for an acute need for aspirin have been published, all with similar rates of success, and all limited in their interpretation by the lack of aspirin challenge to confirm that indeed the patients had aspirin sensitivity in the first place.[26–31] The salient point here is that a patient who is not allergic to aspirin can go through a "desensitization protocol" without "any reaction" and end up taking aspirin in the alleged "desensitized state." For example, Wong and colleagues[27] evaluated 11 patients who required aspirin in the acute setting. The patients mostly had aspirin-associated cutaneous symptoms, although one patient may have had AERD based on the history provided. Rossini and colleagues[28] evaluated 26 patients with acute coronary disease and a history of aspirin allergy. Twenty-three of these patients underwent successful desensitization, but very little of their history of a prior reaction is reported in the article, and no patients had previously undergone a blinded aspirin challenge to confirm they were allergic to aspirin. Two of the 3 patients in whom desensitization was unsuccessful had chronic urticaria worsened by the ingestion of an NSAID. In total, the literature reports 214 patients who underwent aspirin desensitization in an acute setting.[6–14] Desensitization was judged to be "successful" in 203 patients. However, the authors' interpretation is that most of these patients actually underwent negative challenges, and therefore may not have been aspirin sensitive. Five of the 11 failures were in patients with preexisting chronic urticaria. Very importantly, there were no significant complications or morbidity associated with any of the desensitization failures despite the variety of protocols used.

## SCRIPPS CLINIC EXPERIENCE WITH ASPIRIN CHALLENGES AND DESENSITIZATION FOR CAD

Given the lack of compelling data that true IgE-mediated/anaphylactic reactions to aspirin occur, it is likely that prolonged desensitization protocols starting at extremely low doses of aspirin are unnecessary. This notion is in line with the authors' clinical experience at Scripps Clinic over the past 15 years. In an initial evaluation of 30 patients with "aspirin allergy," 24 had a history of urticaria and 6 had a history of anaphylaxis to one NSAID (patients with AERD are not included in this analysis). In the urticaria group, urticaria was due to NSAIDs in 15 patients and due to aspirin in 6. All 6 cases of reported anaphylaxis events were associated with NSAIDs. None were attributed to aspirin. All patients underwent an aspirin challenge starting at 30 mg or 60 mg, based on the preference of the treating physician. None of the 15 patients with NSAID-associated anaphylaxis were challenged with the suspect NSAID. Doses of aspirin were doubled every 30 to 90 minutes until a full 325 mg of aspirin was administered. Twenty-eight patients had a negative challenge, including all 15 patients with prior reactions to other NSAIDs. Of the 6 cases with a prior history of urticaria, after ingesting aspirin 2 patients experienced mild urticaria. Both progressed with successful desensitization to aspirin and continued taking aspirin on a daily basis. There were no cases of anaphylaxis. All were successfully treated with aspirin.

In a more recent case series, 11 patients referred to the authors for "aspirin allergy" and the need for aspirin treatment were evaluated. All underwent aspirin challenge with a starting aspirin dose of either 30 or 40 mg, and the dose was doubled in

90 minutes. One patient had itching, rhinorrhea, and tearing after the second dose was given. This reaction was easily treated with antihistamines, and the final dose of 325 mg was given to ensure that desensitization was complete. One patient developed 2 small hives after the last dose. No patients reacted to the first dose, and in 9 patients there were no objective signs of a reaction. In all patients, a 325-mg dose concluded the challenge, but patients may have been subsequently treated with lower doses of aspirin at the discretion of their other health care providers.

## A PRACTICAL APPROACH TO PATIENTS WITH A HISTORY SUGGESTING ASPIRIN HYPERSENSITIVITY

A practical approach to the urgent need for aspirin administration in the patient with a history of an adverse reaction to aspirin or another NSAID is presented. These recommendations are guided both by an exhaustive review of the literature, and the authors' clinical experience framed by an understanding of the mechanisms of the various aspirin/NSAID reactions.

### The Goal of Aspirin Challenge/Desensitization

In almost all settings, the urgent need for aspirin is necessitated by its well-known antiplatelet effect. Because a significant antiplatelet effect is seen at 81 mg of aspirin, the initial goal of reaching this dose is reasonable for most patients. As seen in the CURRENT-OASIS 7 trial, there was no significant difference in end points between the low dose (75–100 mg aspirin dose) and high dose (300–325 mg daily aspirin) on cardiovascular death, myocardial infarction, and stroke at 30 days.[32] Thus, the goal of the allergist should be to achieve a dose of 81 mg aspirin as quickly and safely as possible. In combination with new potent platelet inhibitors such as prasugrel and clopidogrel, there are no data to suggest that 325 mg of aspirin is more efficacious than 81 mg at preventing restenosis in the first 24 to 48 hours.

The first step in evaluating these patients is to determine whether there is a likelihood of a real aspirin allergy or if they merely have intolerance. Many patients experience side effects such as tinnitus, easy bruisability, or gastrointestinal symptoms, which they attribute to an aspirin allergy. Such patients can be given aspirin without any special protocol.

Once it has been determined that the historical reaction may represent an aspirin allergy, the next step is to characterize the type of reaction (mucocutaneous vs AERD). Every attempt should be made to identify AERD and to obtain historical evidence as to whether a history of reactions or tolerance to any other NSAID exists.

### Location and Timing

The authors believe that for all patients with an unstable arterial lesion (evolving myocardial infarction, evolving transient ischemic attack or cerebrovascular accident, and so forth), the intravascular intervention should occur first and considerations for challenge/desensitization should be secondary. This approach is predicated by the concern that in any patient, there is a real possibility of causing asthma or histamine-mediated coronary vasospasm, which in an already unstable patient could be catastrophic.

The location of the aspirin challenge/desensitization will vary depending on the nursing and monitoring resources available to the allergist. A one-to-one, constant nursing attendance is required, with the supervising physician immediately available. Modalities to treat potentially severe asthmatic and urticarial reactions must be available, including epinephrine. In the authors' institution almost all desensitization/oral challenge procedures occur in the outpatient clinic. Patients discharged soon after cardiac stenting are sent directly to the Allergy outpatient clinic for aspirin challenge and desensitization to aspirin if required. Nevertheless, it is recognized that in other clinics/practices this same approach to aspirin challenge/desensitization will be undertaken in a monitored hospital bed.

In a patient unstable enough that continued hospitalization is necessary for management of the underlying medical condition, the goal of successful aspirin administration is paramount and takes precedence over obtaining an accurate diagnostic aspirin challenge. For this reason, pretreatment with steroids, antihistamines, and montelukast should be considered in all such patients, with the caveat that in a heavily premedicated patient, the lack of any symptoms during the challenge/desensitization procedure cannot be interpreted as a true "negative challenge" but could also represent a "silent desensitization/challenge." This aspect has implications for future aspirin use if there is a lapse in aspirin administration.

The authors believe that the converse situation is true in patients who are stable for discharge from the hospital before aspirin challenge/desensitization. Nearly all of these patients referred to the clinic after hospitalizations can be desensitized in the outpatient setting. In this setting, obtaining an accurate diagnosis is important and can safely be obtained by withholding steroid and antihistamine pretreatment, and by only using these as treatment modalities for patients who react.

### Aspirin Challenge/Desensitization Protocol

Two very similar protocols can be considered, depending on the suspicion of the type of previous reaction (**Fig. 2**).

### AERD

Patients who are asthmatic should be screened for the likelihood of AERD. Many times the patient's history and reported recent tolerance of another NSAID can eliminate the possibility of AERD. With an equivocal history or uncertainty about the diagnosis, further evaluation for AERD should take place. This assessment can be done by performing a nasal examination for polyps and obtaining a Waters view sinus radiograph or computed tomography of the sinuses. If the sinuses are clear or a unilateral opacified sinus is identified, the patient does not have AERD. With pansinusitis, even without prior exposure to aspirin, approximately one-third will have a respiratory reaction to aspirin, signaling the final quatrad of AERD (pansinusitis, nasal polyps, asthma, and aspirin-induced respiratory reaction).

For unstable patients that likely have AERD, the approach is as follows. Pretreatment with oral montelukast 10 mg, inhaled corticosteroid/long-acting β-agonist, systemic corticosteroids (usually intravenous), and antihistamines should be given to everyone. Then, using a pill cutter, give one-half of an 81-mg aspirin tablet. This dose is generally lower than the provoking dose of 60 to 90 mg that causes reactions in most AERD patients. This dose can then be repeated in 90 minutes. At this point the patient will have 81 mg of aspirin in the system, and this 81-mg dose can be repeated daily. In AERD patients, it is likely that they will react to the second dose of 40.5 mg of aspirin. Symptoms will generally be mild to moderate, but should be anticipated and promptly treated with nebulized β-agonists, oral or intravenous antihistamines, or other medications. A thorough review of the treatment or AERD reactions has been published.[33] If a reaction occurs after the first or second dose of aspirin, further dosing the following day should lead to minimal or no further symptoms. At a dose of 81 mg per day some patients may not be completely desensitized, and care should be taken with higher doses of aspirin or other full-strength NSAIDs. In a stable outpatient AERD

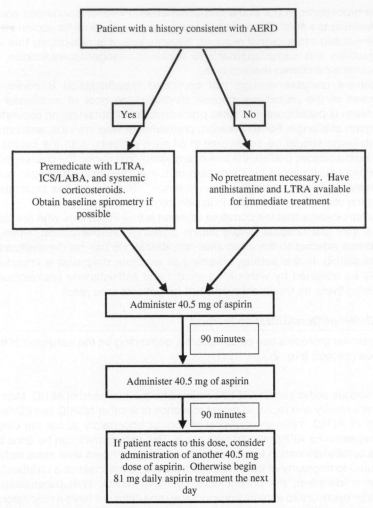

Patient with a history consistent with AERD

Yes

No

Premedicate with LTRA, ICS/LABA, and systemic corticosteroids. Obtain baseline spirometry if possible

No pretreatment necessary. Have antihistamine and LTRA available for immediate treatment

Administer 40.5 mg of aspirin

90 minutes

Administer 40.5 mg of aspirin

90 minutes

If patient reacts to this dose, consider administration of another 40.5 mg dose of aspirin. Otherwise begin 81 mg daily aspirin treatment the next day

**Fig. 2.** Oral aspirin challenge/desensitization algorithm and protocol. AERD, aspirin-exacerbated respiratory disease; ICS, inhaled corticosteroids; LABA, long-acting β2-antagonists; LTRA, leukotriene receptor antagonists.

desensitization, systemic corticosteroids may not be necessary, and antihistamine use as pretreatment may mask symptoms of a reaction and create confusion over whether the patient truly has AERD. It should be noted that at 81 mg a day, the underlying AERD is not going to be treated.

### Cutaneous reactions

Challenge or desensitization can be started at the same doses (40.5 mg aspirin). Pretreatment with an antihistamine and/or leukotriene receptor antagonist is likely to confuse negative versus positive reactions, but these should be added as soon as a cutaneous reaction occurs. A 40.5-mg dose of aspirin is appropriate, and as per the aforementioned protocol can be repeated in 90 minutes to reach the 81-mg target dose. This recommended challenge/desensitization protocol is predicated on the following premise. Conclusive evidence that aspirin can induce IgE-mediated anaphylaxis remains elusive and may not even exist. However, if the presenting patient gives a history of, or emergency-room records document a particularly severe prior aspirin reaction, starting with 20.25 mg of aspirin or less can be considered. Starting with an 81-mg aspirin tablet, a pill cutter can be used to obtain the 20.25-mg dose. In those patients with a severe historical reaction to aspirin, evaluation for AERD is warranted.

With oral desensitizations that involve the hospital pharmacy, there can be a considerable delay in obtaining the required dilutions. In the authors' experience, the majority of patients with a prior cutaneous reaction to another NSAID or a rash occurring more than 10 years previously and associated with ingesting aspirin will not react to 81 mg of aspirin. Conversely, as published recently by McMullan and Wedner,[25] historical reactions to aspirin within the past year are likely to be associated with a reaction during the procedure.

In summary, the approach to the patient with a previous aspirin reaction is to administer half of a baby aspirin (40.5 mg) and repeat the dose in 90 minutes. Only differences in the character of the reaction need to be considered by the ordering physician.

### Proceeding to 325 mg Aspirin

Depending on the intervention, aspirin doses as high as 325 mg may be recommended by the referring cardiologist for optimum antiplatelet effect.[8] This dose can be achieved by continuing the aspirin dosing. Conversely, the patient may be discharged from the acute hospitalization on 81 mg of aspirin, and a follow-up visit may be made to increase the dose to 325 mg. For all patients who have been taking 81 mg aspirin uneventfully, they can undergo the rest of the challenge/desensitization in one visit to the outpatient clinic (see **Fig. 2**).

### Patients Who Should Not be Desensitized to Aspirin

Nearly all patients with a history of a reaction to aspirin will be able to be properly evaluated and treated with aspirin following an oral challenge or desensitization. In a few circumstances the challenge/desensitization or challenge is contraindicated. If there is a history of aspirin-associated Stevens-Johnson syndrome, toxic epidermal necrolysis, hypersensitivity pneumonitis, or drug rash with eosinophilia and systemic symptoms (DRESS) syndrome, rechallenge can be dangerous and desensitization would be unsuccessful. Aspirin is an unlikely candidate for these reactions under any circumstances. In a patient who develops one of these conditions and who has been on a stable dose of aspirin 81 mg a day for years, the culprit drug is more likely to be the newly introduced drug (anticonvulsant, sulfonamide, certain NSAIDs). The problem is that there is a tendency for physicians to stop all medications, even the innocent bystanders. Rechallenge with aspirin, after informed consent, can be considered in this latter circumstance.

Assuming linkage with aspirin, allergic interstitial nephritis and serum sickness will not be amenable to desensitization.[12] Patients with chronic urticarial and historical reactions to aspirin and NSAIDs represent a unique situation. Although desensitization can be safely attempted, in the authors' experience persistent recalcitrant urticaria and angioedema make long-term use of aspirin or NSAIDs very difficult. There is a report of one successful desensitization protocol used for a patient with chronic urticaria requiring aspirin, but this case study cannot be extrapolated to all patients with chronic hives.[34] For patients with chronic urticaria/angioedema with no historical reaction to aspirin, about two-thirds will tolerate aspirin, and it would be appropriate to give them the full dose of 81 mg or 325 mg.

## SUMMARY

With rare exceptions, patients with a history of "aspirin/NSAID allergy" will be able to safely take aspirin after either graded dose challenge or desensitization. Such an inexpensive and effective medication should not be withheld from most patients. A variety of protocols has been described, and although the exact mechanism of desensitization and patient characterization remains somewhat obscure, the take-home message is that in nearly all patients, negative challenge or desensitization was successful. Allergists should be proactive and consistent in their message that aspirin challenge/desensitization can be performed in the acute setting when clinically essential.

## REFERENCES

1. Antithrombotic Trialists Collaboration. Collaborative meta-analysis of randomised trials of antiplatelet therapy for prevention of death, myocardial infarction, and stroke in high risk patients. BMJ 2002;324:71–86.
2. Ryan TJ, Antman EM, Brooks NH, et al. 1999 update: ACC/AHA Guidelines for the Management of Patients With Acute Myocardial Infarction: Executive Summary and Recommendations: a report of the American College of Cardiology/American Heart Association Task Force on Practice Guidelines (Committee on Management of Acute Myocardial Infarction). Circulation 1999;100:1016–30.
3. Braunwald E, Antman EM, Beasley JW, et al. ACC/AHA guidelines for the management of patients with unstable angina and non-ST-segment elevation myocardial infarction: executive summary and recommendations. A report of the American College of Cardiology/American Heart Association task force on practice guidelines (committee on the management of patients with unstable angina). Circulation 2000;102:1193–209.
4. Sabatine MS, Cannon CP, Gibson CM, et al. Addition of clopidogrel to aspirin and fibrinolytic therapy for myocardial infarction with ST-segment elevation. N Engl J Med 2005;352:1179–89.
5. Yusuf S, Zhao F, Mehta SR, et al. Effects of clopidogrel in addition to aspirin in patients with acute coronary syndromes without ST-segment elevation. N Engl J Med 2001;345:494–502.
6. Mehta SR, Yusuf S, Peters RJ, et al. Effects of pretreatment with clopidogrel and aspirin followed by long-term therapy in patients undergoing percutaneous coronary intervention: the PCI-CURE study. Lancet 2001;358:527–33.
7. Steinhubl SR, Berger PB, Mann JT 3rd, et al. Early and sustained dual oral antiplatelet therapy following percutaneous coronary intervention: a randomized controlled trial. JAMA 2002;288:2411–20.
8. Smith SC Jr, Feldman TE, Hirshfeld JW Jr, et al. ACC/AHA/SCAI 2005 guideline update for percutaneous coronary intervention: a report of the American College of Cardiology/American Heart Association Task Force on Practice Guidelines (ACC/AHA/SCAI Writing Committee to Update 2001 Guidelines for Percutaneous Coronary Intervention). Circulation 2006;113:e166–286.
9. Gaspoz JM, Coxson PG, Goldman PA, et al. Cost effectiveness of aspirin, clopidogrel, or both for secondary prevention of coronary heart disease. N Engl J Med 2002;346:1800–6.
10. Settipane RA, Constantine HP, Settipane GA. Aspirin intolerance and recurrent urticaria in normal adults and children. Epidemiology and review. Allergy 1980;35:149–54.
11. Gomes E, Cardoso MF, Praca F, et al. Self-reported drug allergy in a general adult Portuguese population. Clin Exp Allergy 2004;34:1597–601.

12. Kowalski ML, Makowska JS, Blanca M, et al. Hypersensitivity to nonsteroidal anti-inflammatory drugs (NSAIDs)—classification, diagnosis and management: review of the EAACI/ENDA(#) and GA2LEN/HANNA*. Allergy 2011;66:818–29.
13. Hedman J, Kaprio J, Poussa T, et al. Prevalence of asthma, aspirin intolerance, nasal polyposis and chronic obstructive pulmonary disease in a population-based study. Int J Epidemiol 1999;28:717–22.
14. Jenkins C, Costello J, Hodge L. Systematic review of prevalence of aspirin induced asthma and its implications for clinical practice. BMJ 2004;328:434.
15. Moore-Robinson M, Warin RP. Effect of salicylates in urticaria. Br Med J 1967;4:262–4.
16. Solensky R. Drug allergy: desensitization and treatment of reactions to antibiotics and aspirin. In: Lockey P, editor. Allergens and allergen immunotherapy. New York: Marcel Dekker; 2004. p. 585–606.
17. Szczeklik A, Nizankowska-Mogilnicka E, Sanak M. Hypersensitivity to aspirin and non-steroidal anti-inflammatory drugs. In: Adkinson NF, Bochner BS, Busse WW, et al, editors. Middleton's allergy: principles and practice. Philadelphia: Mosby; 2008. p. 1227–39.
18. Grattan CE. Aspirin sensitivity and urticaria. Clin Exp Dermatol 2003;28:123–7.
19. Mathison DA, Lumry WR, Stevenson DD. Aspirin in chronic urticaria and/or angioedema: studies of sensitivity and desensitization. J Allergy Clin Immunol 1982;69:135.
20. Doeglas HM. Reactions to aspirin and food additives in patients with chronic urticaria, including the physical urticarias. Br J Dermatol 1975;93:135–44.
21. Kemp SF, Lockey RF, Wolf BL, et al. Anaphylaxis. A review of 266 cases. Arch Intern Med 1995;155:1749–54.
22. Phills JA, Perelmutter L. IgE mediated and non-IgE mediated allergic-type reactions to aspirin. Acta Allergol 1974;29:474–90.
23. Blanca M, Perez E, Garcia JJ, et al. Angioedema and IgE antibodies to aspirin: a case report. Ann Allergy 1989;62:295–8.
24. De Luca G, Verdoia M, Binda G, et al. Aspirin desensitization in patients undergoing planned or urgent coronary stent implantation. A single-center experience. Int J Cardiol 2012. [Epub ahead of print].
25. McMullan KL, Wedner HJ. Safety of aspirin desensitization in patients with reported aspirin allergy and cardiovascular disease. Clin Cardiol 2012. [Epub ahead of print].
26. Fajt ML, Petrov AA. Outpatient aspirin desensitization for patients with aspirin hypersensitivity and cardiac disease. Crit Pathw Cardiol 2011;10:17–21.
27. Wong JT, Nagy CS, Krinzman SJ, et al. Rapid oral challenge-desensitization for patients with aspirin-related urticaria-angioedema. J Allergy Clin Immunol 2000;105:997–1001.
28. Rossini R, Angiolillo DJ, Musumeci G, et al. Aspirin desensitization in patients undergoing percutaneous coronary interventions with stent implantation. Am J Cardiol 2008;101:786–9.
29. Dalmau G, Gaig P, Gazquez V, et al. Rapid desensitization to acetylsalicylic acid in acute coronary syndrome patients with NSAID intolerance. Rev Esp Cardiol 2009;02.224–5.
30. Silberman S, Neukirch-Stoop C, Steg PG. Rapid desensitization procedure for patients with aspirin hypersensitivity undergoing coronary stenting. Am J Cardiol 2005;95:509–10.
31. Ortega-Loayza AG, Raza S, Minisi AJ, et al. Aspirin desensitization/challenge in 3 patients with unstable angina. Am J Med Sci 2010;340:418–20.

32. Mehta SR, Tanguay JF, Eikelboom JW, et al. Double-dose versus standard-dose clopidogrel and high-dose versus low-dose aspirin in individuals undergoing percutaneous coronary intervention for acute coronary syndromes (CURRENT-OASIS 7): a randomised factorial trial. Lancet 2010;376:1233–43.

33. Stevenson DD, Simon RA. Selection of patients for aspirin desensitization treatment. J Allergy Clin Immunol 2006;118:801–4.

34. Slowik SM, Slavin RG. Aspirin desensitization in a patient with aspirin sensitivity and chronic idiopathic urticaria. Ann Allergy Asthma Immunol 2009;102:171–2.

# Index

*Note:* Page numbers of article titles are in **boldface** type.

### A

Abdominal pain, 137–138
Acetaminophen, respiratory reactions to, 150
Acetylsalicylic acid. *See also* Aspirin.
   development of, 135–136
*ACORA3* gene, in hypersensitivity, 185–186
Acute generalized exanthematous pustulosis, 242
Adenosine, in hypersensitivity, 186
AECD. *See* Aspirin-exacerbated cutaneous disease (urticaria and angioedema).
AERD. *See* Aspirin-exacerbated respiratory disease.
*ALOX5* gene, in hypersensitivity, 178–179, 184
Anaphylaxis, 138, 238–240
Angioedema. *See* Aspirin-exacerbated cutaneous disease (urticaria and angioedema).
Angiotensin-converting enzyme, in hypersensitivity, 183–186
Angiotensinogen, in hypersensitivity, 183, 185
Antibiotics, for rhinosinusitis and nasal polyps, 171
Antihistamines, for AECD, 258–259
Antipyrine, 135–136
Arachidonic acid, metabolism of, 136–137
   desensitization and, 225–227
   genetic studies of, 178–179
   in rhinosinusitis with nasal polyps, 166–169
   pathogenesis and, 199–202
Aseptic meningitis, 244
Aspirin
   for cardiovascular prophylaxis, **263–274**
   history of, 135–137
   metabolism of, genetic factors in, 186
   pharmacology of, 224–225
   provocation tests with, for AERD, 152–157
Aspirin desensitization
   contraindications to, 271
   for AERD, **211–222**
      alternative antiinflammatory effects of, 231–232
      arachidonic acid metabolites and, 225–227
      current practices in, 217–220
      early effects of, 215
      efficacy of, 213–215
      eosinophil responses after, 230–231
      history of, 211–213

http://dx.doi.org/10.1016/S0889-8561(13)00026-X

Aspirin (*continued*)
    interleukin alterations after, 228–230
    leukotriene receptor expression and, 227–228
    mast cell response after, 230–231
    mechanisms of, **223–236**
    medications with, 215–217
    safety of, 213–214
  for cardiovascular prophylaxis, 268–271
  for rhinosinusitis and nasal polyps, 171–172
"Aspirin triad," 140, 148
Aspirin-exacerbated cutaneous disease (urticaria and angioedema), 238–240, **251–262**
  cardiovascular prophylaxis and, 265–266, 270–271
  clinical features of, 254–255
  definition of, 142, 252–253
  diagnosis of, 255–258
  first cases of, 140–141
  pathogenesis of, 253–254
  pharmacology of, 252
  prevalence of, 252–253
  prognosis for, 255
  treatment of, 258–260
Aspirin-exacerbated respiratory disease, **147–161**
  cardiovascular prophylaxis and, 265, 269–270
  clinical presentation of, 149–150
  definition of, 142, 147–148
  desensitization in, 171–172, **211–236**
  diagnosis of, **147–161,** 152–157
  first cases of, 140
  history of, 148
  natural history of, 148
  pathogenesis of, **195–210**
    cyclooxygenase pathway in, 199–202
    histopathology, 196–197
    lipid mediators in, 197–199
  prevalence of, 148
  rhinosinusitis with nasal polyps in, **163–175**
  sinonasal manifestations in, **163–175**
  types of NSAIDs causing, 150–151
Aspirin-Sensitive Patients Identification Test, 170
ASPIT test, for AERD, 157
Asthma, in AERD, 148–150
Autoimmunity, AECD and, 254
Avoidance, for rhinosinusitis and nasal polyps, 170


**B**

Basophil activation test, for AERD, 157
Beers, R. F., 140
Bleeding, 138
Bullous cutaneous reactions, severe, 242–243

**C**

*CACNG6* gene, in hypersensitivity, 183
Calcium-signaling pathway, in hypersensitivity, 183, 185
Candidate gene studies, of hypersensitivity, 178–181
Cardiovascular prophylaxis
   with aspirin hypersensitive
      approach to, 268–271
      efficacy of, 263–265
      literature review for, 266–267
      reaction types and, 265–266
      Scripps experience with, 267–268
   with aspirin hypersensitivity, **263–274**
Carprofen, chemical structure of, 138
*CCR3* gene, in hypersensitivity, 180
Celecoxib
   cardiac toxicity of, 245
   respiratory reactions to, 150–151
*CEP68* gene, in hypersensitivity, 181
Chemokines, in hypersensitivity, 180, 185
Computed tomography, for rhinosinusitis with nasal polyps, 169
Contact dermatitis, 244
Corticosteroids
   for AECD, 258
   for asthma, 149
   for rhinosinusitis and nasal polyps, 170
*COX-1* gene, in hypersensitivity, 178–179
*CRTH2* gene, in hypersensitivity, 180
Cutaneous diseases. *See* Aspirin-exacerbated cutaneous disease (urticaria and angioedema).
Cyclooxygenase
   in AERD, 202–205
   in rhinosinusitis with nasal polyps, 166–168
   inhibition of, 136–137, 141
Cyclooxygenase-1 inhibitors, respiratory reactions to, 150–151
Cyclooxygenase-2 inhibitors
   cardiac toxicity of, 245
   respiratory reactions to, 150–151
Cyclosporine, for AECD, 258
*CYSLTR* genes, in hypersensitivity, 178, 184
Cytochrome P450, in hypersensitivity, 185–186
Cytokines, in rhinosinusitis with nasal polyps, 165–166


**D**

Dermatitis, 244
Desensitization, aspirin. *See* Aspirin desensitization.
DRESS syndrome (drug rash with eosinophilia and systemic symptoms), 243–244


**E**

Effector function, of inflammatory cells, genetic studies of, 179–181
*EMID2* gene, in hypersensitivity, 182, 184

ENFUMOSA study, 149
Eosinophils
    in AERD, 196
    in aspirin desensitization, 230–231
    in rhinosinusitis with nasal polyps, 165
Eoxins, in hypersensitivity, 179
Epigenetics, in hypersensitivity, 187
Epithelial cell dysfunction, in hypersensitivity, 182–183
Ethmoidotomy, for rhinosinusitis and nasal polyps, 171


F

*FCER1A* gene, in hypersensitivity, 180
*FFPR1* gene, in hypersensitivity, 179
Fixed drug eruptions, 242
Flurbiprofen, chemical structure of, 138
Functional endoscopic sinus surgery, for rhinosinusitis and nasal polyps, 171


G

Gamma-aminiobutyric acid, in hypersensitivity, 183
Gastritis, 137–138
Gene-gene interactions, in hypersensitivity, 186–187
Genetic studies, of hypersensitivity, **177–194**
    historical review of, 178–181
    limitations of, 186–187
    present knowledge of, 181–186
Genome-wide association studies, of hypersensitivity, 181
Gilbert, G. B., 140
Granulocytes, in AERD, 196


H

Heart, NSAID toxicity to, 245
Hirschberg, Doctor, 140
Hives. *See* Aspirin-exacerbated respiratory disease.
*HNMT* gene, in hypersensitivity, 180, 185
Hoffman, Felix, 135–136, 224
Human leukocyte antigens
    in AECD, 254
    in hypersensitivity, 181–182, 184
15-Hydroxyeicosanoic acid generation assay, for AERD, 157
15-Hydroxyeicsoatetranoic acid, in hypersensitivity, 179
Hypersensitivity pneumonitis, 244
Hypersensitivity reactions, 139–140. *See also specific reactions.*
    classification of, 140–141
    definitions of, 142
    diagnosis of, 142–144
    first cases of, 140
    subtypes of, 141
    to single drugs, **237–249**

acute, 238, 240
classification of, 238–239
delayed, 240–244
diagnosis of, 240, 245
treatment of, 245


I

Ibuprofen
chemical structure of, 138
discovery of, 136
respiratory reactions to, 150
IL1RL1 gene, in hypersensitivity, 181
Immune response, initiation of, in hypersensitivity, 182
Immunosuppressive agents, for AECD, 258
Indomethacin, discovery of, 136
Inflammation, signaling of, in hypersensitivity, 183, 186
Inflammatory cells, effector function of, genetic studies of, 179–181
Inhalation provocation tests, for AERD, 154–156, 169–170
Interleukins
in aspirin desensitization, 228–230
in hypersensitivity, 180, 185


K

Ketoprofen, chemical structure of, 138
Ketorolac
for aspirin desensitization, 219
respiratory reactions to, 150
KIF3A gene, in hypersensitivity, 182–184
Kinesins, in hypersensitivity, 182–184
Knorr, Ludwig, 135–136


L

Leukotriene(s)
in AERD, 197–200
in aspirin desensitization, 225–228
in hypersensitivity, 178–180, 184
in rhinosinusitis with nasal polyps, 166–169
Leukotriene inhibitors
for aspirin desensitization, 216–217
for rhinosinusitis and nasal polyps, 171
Leukotriene receptor antagonists, 178
5-Lipooxygenase, in hypersensitivity, 178
Lipoxins
in AERD, 202
in aspirin desensitization, 227
in hypersensitivity, 179
Lipoxygenase pathway, in arachidonic acid metabolism, 168–169

## M

Maculopapular exanthems, 240–242
Mast cells
  in AERD, 196
  in aspirin desensitization, 230–231
  in hypersensitivity, 180
  in rhinosinusitis with nasal polyps, 165–166
Meloxicam, respiratory reactions to, 150
Meningitis, aseptic, 244
Methylation, in hypersensitivity, 187
Montelukast, for aspirin desensitization, 218–219
Multiple NSAID-induced urticaria/angioedema, definition of, 142

## N

Naproxen
  chemical structure of, 138
  respiratory reactions to, 150
Nasal polyps, 148
  rhinosinusitis with, in AERD, **163–175**
    definitions of, 164
    diagnosis of, 169–170
    epidemiology of, 164–165
    natural history of, 164–165
    pathophysiology of, 165–169
    treatment of, 170–172
Nasal provocation tests, for AERD, 156–157
Nasal reactions, in AERD, 149–150
*NAT* gene, in hypersensitivity, 186
Neutrophils, in hypersensitivity, 180–181
Next-generation sequencing, in hypersensitivity, 187
NFAT transcription factor, in aspirin desensitization, 232
Nimesulide, respiratory reactions to, 150
Nonsteroidal anti-inflammatory drugs. *See also* Aspirin *and individual drugs.*
  chemical structures of, 137
  classification of, by chemical structure, 137
  history of, 135–137
  hypersensitivity to. *See* Hypersensitivity reactions.
  mechanism of action of, 136–137
  pharmacology of, 224–225
  reactions to, 137–140
    classification of, **135–145**
    delayed, 142
    single-drug, **237–249**
    Szczeklik publications on, **125–133**
    type A, 139
    type B, 139
NSAIDs. *See* Nonsteroidal anti-inflammatory drugs.
Nuclear factor-κB, in aspirin desensitization, 231

**O**

Omalizumab, for AECD, 258
1000 Genomes Project, 187
Oral provocation tests, for AERD, 154, 169–170
*ORMDL3* gene, in hypersensitivity, 181
Oxyphenbutazone, chemical structure of, 138


**P**

*PDE4D* gene, in hypersensitivity, 181
Peroxisome proliferator-activated receptors, in hypersensitivity, 183, 185
Phenylbutazone
    chemical structure of, 138
    discovery of, 136
Photoallergic dermatitis, 244
Platelets, in hypersensitivity, 180
Pneumonitis, hypersensitivity, 244
Polypectomy, for rhinosinusitis and nasal polyps, 171
Polyps, nasal. *See* Nasal polyps.
*PPARG* gene, in hypersensitivity, 183, 185
Prostaglandins
    in AERD, 199–204
    in hypersensitivity, 184
    in rhinosinusitis with nasal polyps, 166–168
Prostanoid receptor, in AERD, 201–202
Provocation tests
    for AECD, 257
    for AERD, 152–157
*PTGER2* gene, in hypersensitivity, 178–179, 184
Pustulosis, acute generalized exanthematous, 242


**R**

*RAD50* gene, in hypersensitivity, 181
Rhinosinusitis, with nasal polyps, in AERD, **163–175**
    definitions of, 164
    diagnosis of, 169–170
    epidemiology of, 164–165
    natural history of, 164–165
    pathophysiology of, 165–169
    treatment of, 170–172
Rofecoxib, respiratory reactions to, 150–151


**S**

Saline irrigation, for rhinosinusitis and nasal polyps, 170–171
Samter, Max, 140
Samter's triad, 140, 148

Single NSAID-induced urticaria/angioedema
  cardiovascular prophylaxis and, 266
  definition of, 142
Skin reactions, 138. *See also* Aspirin-exacerbated cutaneous disease; Aspirin-exacerbated
  cutaneous disease (urticaria and angioedema).
*SPINK* gene, in hypersensitivity, 182, 184
Stevens-Johnson syndrome, 242–243
Stevenson, D. D., 141, 213, 224
*STK10* gene, in hypersensitivity, 183, 185
Sulfidoleukotriene release assay, for AERD, 157
Szczeklik, Andrew, **125–133,** 140–141


**T**

*TBXAS* genes, in hypersensitivity, 179, 184
TENOR (The Epidemiology and Natural History of Asthma: Outcomes and Treatment
  Regimens) study, 149
Thromboxanes, in AERD, 199–200
Toxic epidermal necrolysis, 242–243
Transcellular biosynthesis, in arachidonic acid metabolism, 166–167, 169


**U**

Ubiquitin–proteasome pathway-related gene, in hypersensitivity, 183–184
Urticaria. *See* Aspirin-exacerbated cutaneous disease (urticaria and angioedema).
Urticaria and angioedema, genetic factors in, 179


**V**

Vane, John, 136–137, 140, 224
Viral infections, hypersensitivity and, 182


**W**

Widal, M.F., 136, 140, 211–213, 223–224

# *Moving?*

## *Make sure your subscription moves with you!*

To notify us of your new address, find your **Clinics Account Number** (located on your mailing label above your name), and contact customer service at:

**Email: journalscustomerservice-usa@elsevier.com**

**800-654-2452** (subscribers in the U.S. & Canada)
**314-447-8871** (subscribers outside of the U.S. & Canada)

**Fax number: 314-447-8029**

**Elsevier Health Sciences Division
Subscription Customer Service
3251 Riverport Lane
Maryland Heights, MO 63043**

Printed and bound by CPI Group (UK) Ltd, Croydon, CR0 4YY

03/10/2024

01040454-0011